The Method Training Program

Wellness Strategies for Life

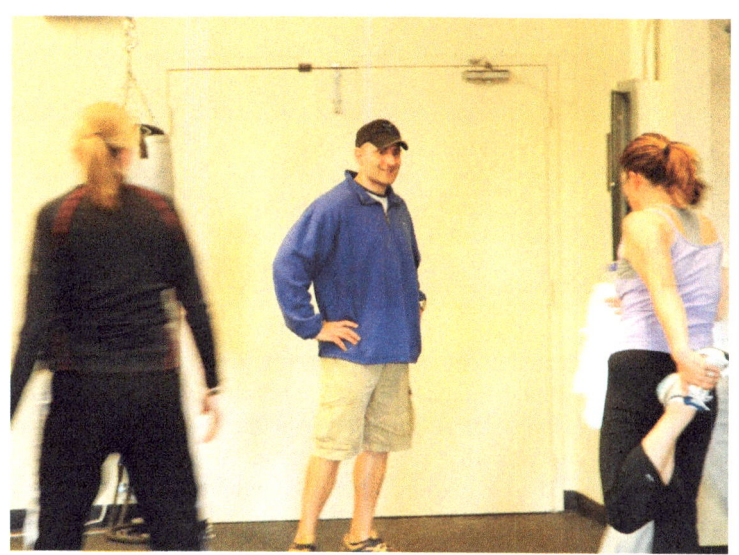

"A wellness plan for anyone that has ever struggled to succeed in fitness."

By *Cody Foss*

Dedication

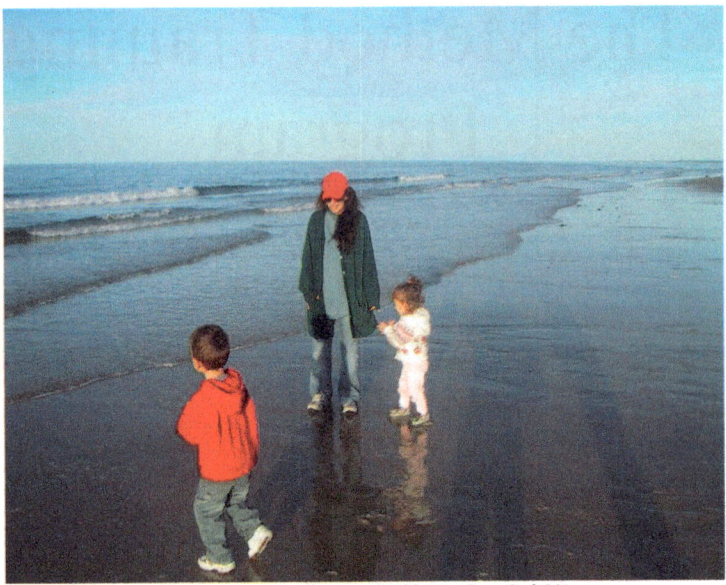

Karen Foss with 2 of her grandchildren in Cape Cod, MA.

This book is dedicated to my mother, Karen Foss. My mother passed away several years ago, but the impact of her life is still very much felt today. She was my greatest supporter and raised me with the belief that anything is possible. My mom was kind and non-judgmental. She saw everyone for their strengths and had empathy and understanding for their shortcomings. She sought to understand people and people would often seek her out for advice as there was no greater person to meet with for a cup of coffee or tea to discuss the problems of the world.

She was a single mother with only a high school education that managed to raise me and at the same time, created an impactful life dedicated to helping others. My mom loved animals, especially dogs, so they played a major part in our lives and were treated like family. She was unique in her belief in animal powers, magic, crystals, and shamans, to name a few. She had her own unique style as well, was a buyer for a high-end clothing store, and developed a knack for showcasing window displays.

However, while fashion was her first recognized talent, her true calling came during the 2nd half of her career when she dedicated herself to helping at-risk youth. As she bravely dealt with her own struggles, she became a counselor focusing on children dealing with drug and alcohol dependency.

She went back to school, after not having advanced past a high school education, and worked extremely hard to obtain the necessary education to become a counselor. My mother, more than any person I've ever known, continued to evolve as a human being over the course of her life. She was not only a true inspiration to me, but to countless people.

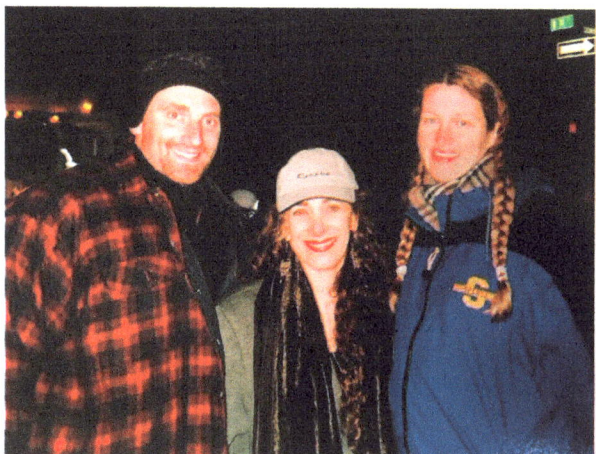
Myself with my wife and mother after the 2002 NYC Marathon.

That inspiration fostered my lifelong goal of one day opening my own gym. One of my proudest moments was opening my gym, The Fitness Loft, while she was still alive. Not only was she able to see me realize my dream, but she was also able to observe the amazing community support and connection we had with our members.

The Fitness Loft was transformational for me as I really began to experience the impact of community. I began to shift away from just helping individuals as I started to appreciate the scale and scope of what wellness really meant. Working together as a group creates a greater impact and these shared experiences forge deep relationships. What started as a career focused on individual training, evolved into wellness opportunities for the community at large. What I learned from The Fitness Loft led me to start wellness initiatives for entire communities; to develop after school programs where children could address mental, physical, and emotional well-being; to develop family-friendly adventure races; and to work for nonprofits addressing social-emotional intelligence as well as physical well-being.

So, while I didn't see it initially, I realize now that I've been (PROUDLY) following in my mother's footsteps. My mother instilled in me that our lives are meant to be spent evolving as human beings and helping others along the way!

Table of Contents

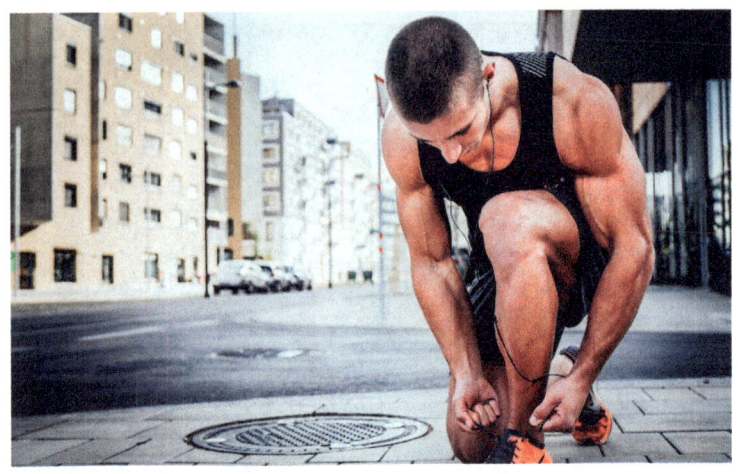

Introduction

Chapter 1: Evolution of The Method

Chapter 2: Why People are Failing at Fitness

Chapter 3: Resting Metabolic Rate

Chapter 4: Cardiovascular Training

Chapter 5: Strength Training

Chapter 6: Caloric Consumption and Nutrition

Chapter 7: Your Crucible

Chapter 8: Connect with Others to Inspire Their Journey

Chapter 9: Mindset

Chapter 10: Building Your Plan

Introduction

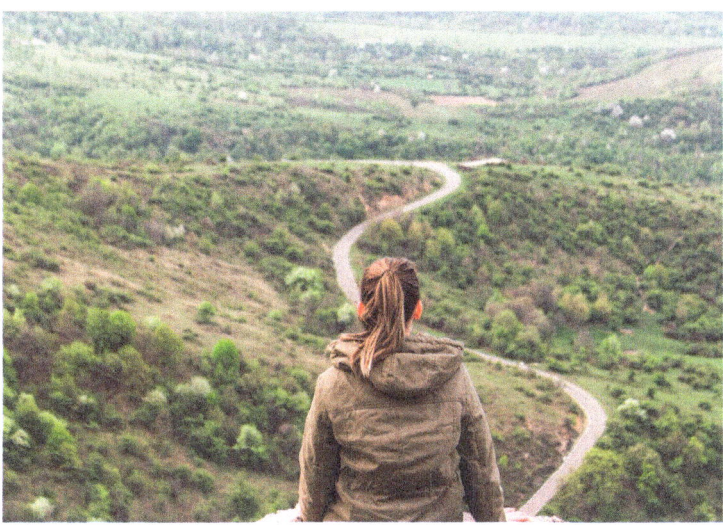

Congratulations on taking the next step to improve your health and wellness! The Method is a scientifically validated program that will customize a wellness plan specifically for you. Your program will be tailored to your strengths and interests and will create opportunities for success driven by proven strategies. I will provide you with the necessary information to succeed and to avoid the missteps that typically sabotage others. The Method will teach you how to build a body that works more functionally for you.

1. Did you realize that if you gain one pound of lean body mass by strength training, you will lose additional pounds over the course of a year from the calories needed to sustain that new muscle?

2. Did you realize that there are certain types of cardiovascular training that will continue to burn calories even after you are done working out?

3. Did you know that certain types of food not only provide your body with necessary nutrients and fuel but will rev up your metabolism, burning calories even while you are not working out?

I've been recognized as an expert in Health and Wellness for almost 30 years and have helped thousands of people achieve success using The Method. Together, we are going to change the message! **It's not what you can't do, it's about what you can do.** We are going to focus on your positive attributes and use them to catapult you into a fitness program and lifestyle that works for you. However, as a warning, if you are looking for a quick, easy fix, then this is not the right program for you. My goal is to empower you to feel better about yourself and to help you take the progressive steps to lead a successful life of health and wellness. I look forward to starting this journey with you and I'm so excited to help you achieve success!

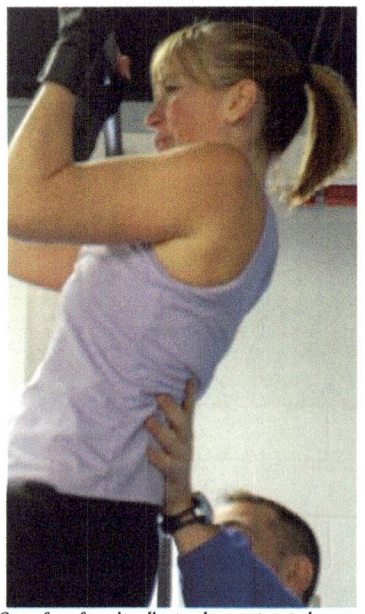

One of my favorite clients who went on to become an amazing personal trainer herself.

Chapter 1:
Evolution of The Method

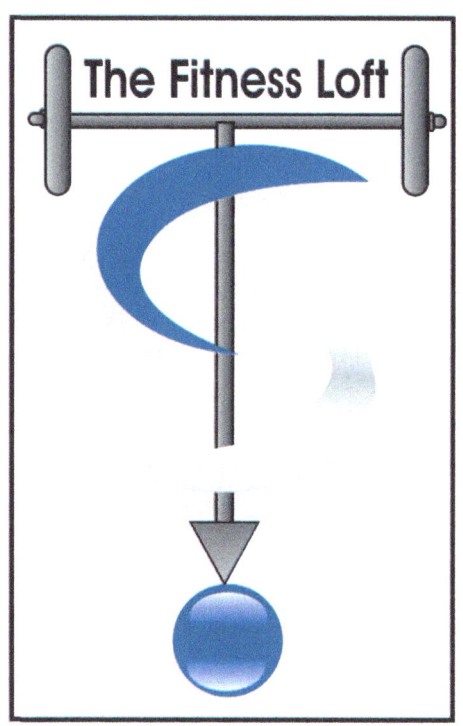

"Passion and Purpose"
When I was in the 6th grade, I bought my first weight set. Motivated by being "chubby", becoming interested in sports and trying to impress my dad, I desperately wanted to get in better shape. Little did I know that I had taken my first step toward a successful career in health and wellness. I was an awkward pre-teen living in the even more awkward eighties, the era of hairbands and the fitness revolution. Images ranged from the hulking Arnold Schwarzenegger to the flamboyant king of cardio, Richard Simmons. Both individuals were deemed experts in the field of fitness, but they held opposing messages, physiques, and philosophies. Beverages like Tab Cola and fat-free products filled our refrigerators and I found myself, like everyone else, a bit confused by what exercises I should do or what food I should eat. Fortunately for me, simple laws of physics and the hormones inherent in becoming a teenager allowed me to reach some level

of success without any real guidance. This success came thanks to the purchase of my first weight set, a cheap barbell set coated in plastic and filled with a weighted substance, presumably concrete. The red covered weights came with a flimsy bench and weight clasps that were supposed to secure the weights to the barbell. Somehow, they never seemed to stay on, regardless of how hard I tightened them. This led to further increased risk of my already questionable workouts. However, no risk was greater than my assumption that the supplemental poster which came with the weight set would provide me all the necessary information and guidance I would need.

Most days after school I would come home and simply workout by myself, trying to mimic the images demonstrated in the exercise poster. My logic was simple, if that guy (model) in the poster did those exercises and looked that good, it had to work for me, right? I realize this might sound dramatic but working out was becoming the one thing in my life that seemed to be fair, consistent, and made sense. If I worked hard, it promised to yield positive results. Unlike other parts of my life like school, girls, and sports, I could control the variables required for fitness. This is where I learned my first very important lesson from fitness. Life is chaotic and filled with constant ebbs and flows, however, **most of us have the ability to control our physical well-being.** So, fitness was working for me, I felt better about the way I looked and a life of wellness was underway. From the day I brought home those weights, my life path and journey changed.

"Supply and demand lead to the creation of The Method"
There is no question my early passion for sports and fitness led to my career path in sports medicine and wellness. I went on to pursue both, obtaining my Master's in Health Sciences and acquiring every significant degree I could get. As I started my career in my early 20's, I had purpose and passion.

However, passion is one thing, being able to deliver results on a consistent basis and being paid for your knowledge and instruction is another. I was very fortunate to obtain measurable success as a personal trainer relatively quickly. My background and the experience I had obtained had allowed me to provide my clients with a very unique training experience. My programs were functional and scientific and were yielding results. I was able to unlock information during assessments that would provide invaluable information to me to provide exercises that would address weaknesses, account for previous injuries, and my clients began to look and feel better. Without realizing it, my philosophy and methodology was the basis for "The Method". What's interesting is that the knowledge required to be a trainer was easy, but for me, the challenge was in developing a business model for growth. My initial concerns about securing enough clients was quickly surpassed by how can I continue to grow my business. Successful trainers very quickly learn the law of supply and demand as you can only fill so many training hours in a day. I initially adjusted my hourly rate, but again, growth was still stymied by the limitations of time. I realized I had to be much more efficient with the total time I spent on each client. The hour spent training the client couldn't be modified, but the time spent planning and modifying their program could be more efficient. So, I began to work on developing a resource that would allow me to capture The Method assessment and program design more systematically. I moved to more automated systems and utilized software like Excel to reduce the time spent on program design (remember my career started in the late 90's, so the technology we currently have available didn't exist).

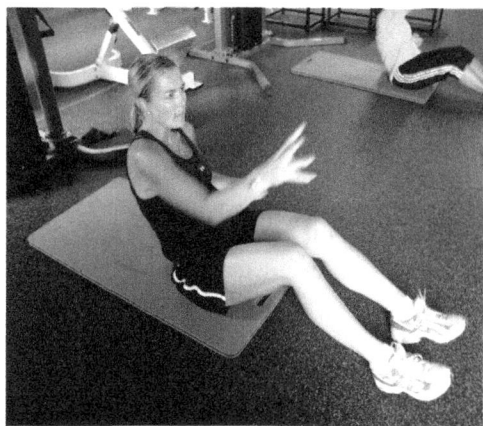

This client arguably achieved the best shape of her life in her 40's.

Once I learned how to better manage a busy training schedule, the next progression in the development of The Method occurred when I opened my own gym in Newtown, CT with my wife in 2006. We were a modest "Mom and Pop Shop", but we had a knowledge base and reputation for members getting great results and this was quickly allowing us to separate ourselves, or our gym, from our competitors.

A major reason for our success was our onboarding for new members, as each of them received a customized assessment and program design as part of their membership. Normally gyms provide a basic assessment and try to sell personal training, we were delivering much more. I personally provided over 300 assessments and programs the first year alone. Every member was exposed to The Method and whether they knew it or not, they were providing me with invaluable data and feedback, which led to continued improvements with this system. This was tremendously satisfying to me as I was able to increase the scale and impact of my training programs and **our gym was providing the personal training effect without requiring personal training!**

Looking back now on the evolution of The Method, this is a tried and proven program with information obtained from higher education, years of experience in developing the program and ultimate proven success in both training personal clients as well as gym members following the program on their own.

"Influence and Inspiration"
As I mentioned in my dedication, I am forever grateful to my mom for what she instilled in me to get to where I am today. Additionally, there are several other significant influences throughout my life that not only helped me individually but impacted the development of The Method.

Coaches
Sports played a major role in my life from youth through college and I was blessed to have countless great coaches along the way. The time, effort, and energy invested in me by these people instilled in me many life lessons and skills that have greatly influenced me both personally and professionally. A large part of success in the health and wellness field is dependent on your personality and how well you can work with others. I believe my social skill set is a positive attribute and was impacted and shaped by the coaches in my life. Of the countless coaches that I could acknowledge, my youth football coach, Buddy Jobin, and my high school football coach, Ed Mantie, stand out the most.

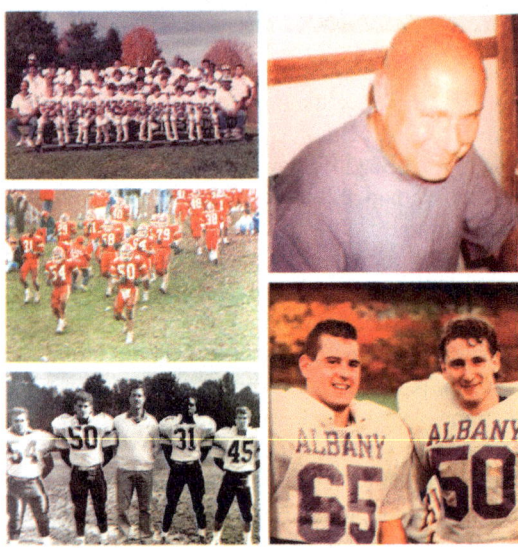

*Top right: Buddy Jobin. Bottom left: Coach Mantie (in between his 4 captains).
Also featured are teammates from youth thru college football*

"Buddy" was a volunteer coach that ran the Maroon Youth Football Program in my hometown of Mount Kisco, NY. He was a sanitation worker by day and a tough, hard-nosed coach with a heart of gold in the afternoons. Buddy was less of a tactician and more of a gritty motivator, but he loved his community and the athletes that played for him. Like so many athletes before and after me, I knew he genuinely cared about me and I was a better player and person for being coached by him. Buddy was my first example of the impact that **volunteering to serve your community** can have.

Coach Mantie was an unbelievably successful high school coach whose claim to fame, other than his dominant run as The Fox Lane Foxes Head Coach, was being the roommate and teammate of NFL Hall of Famer, Larry Csonka, while they both attended Syracuse University. Coach Mantie was a meticulous planner and tactician. He always assembled a great coaching staff and the details in his preparation were a key contributor to his success. Coach Mantie was a father figure to a lot of kids in his program, but his commitment to his own family was always present. In fact, Coach Mantie walked away from coaching at the peak of his career to watch his son, Ed Jr, play in their hometown of Danbury, CT. Coach Mantie taught me the value of **preparation and discipline to achieve the desired outcome.**

I hope both coaches know how grateful I am and that I'm doing my best to follow in their footsteps as a volunteer youth coach in my community.

Professional Colleagues
In addition to my coaches, I've been blessed to work with many talented colleagues who taught me so much about sports medicine and wellness. Most notably, I must credit a friend of mine, Alwyn Cosgrove, who over the years has taught me more about the **fitness business and creating effective training systems** than anyone. Alwyn and I worked together in the late 90's at a cutting edge physical therapy and performance center in NYC called the US Athletic Training Center (USATC).

We were fortunate enough to be mentored by the owner, Gary Guerrero. Gary combined his extensive background as a physical therapist, athletic trainer, and strength coach to aggressively implement results-driven therapeutic and performance training strategies for both athletes and the general population. Gary was a demanding employer and made it clear that if you wanted to keep your job, you needed to understand and be capable of implementing his methodology and protocols. Gary's principles were founded in science and he pushed all of us to fully understand the anatomy and physiology of the body at higher levels than what was required through traditional education. Gary **believed that science was at the route of every decision we made** and if you wanted to offer a suggestion, you had to be able to justify it through science. Working at the USATC was an exciting time professionally as Gary had established himself as a sought-out expert and was involved with training Olympic and professional athletes.

Gary assembled a blend of independent trainers along with the USATC performance team to work together to form a super talented staff.

Fortunately for me at this time, a friend, Steve Didio, and I were getting our Master's in Health Sciences together and Steve was the manager at the USATC. Steve brought me into the fold of this amazing team and provided me with an opportunity that shaped my career forever. Steve has since gone on to own and manage several training facilities in Westchester, NY. In addition to Alwyn and Steve, there was also Ben Velasquez, Mike Mejia, Darren Vella, Spencer Marcus, Dan Owens, to name a few, all of which have had accomplished careers. However, in my opinion, Alwyn was the most talented of the group and it was inevitable that he would establish the career that he has. Alwyn is recognized as one of the most knowledgeable trainers in the industry and is nationally recognized for his training systems and business expertise in the world of fitness.

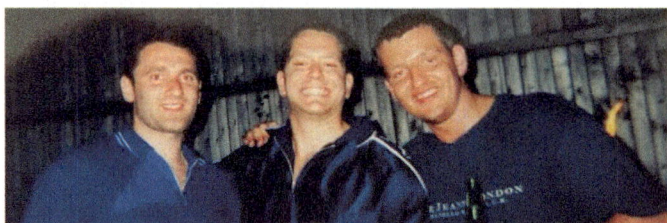

Left to right: myself, Steve Didio and Alwyn Cosgrove.

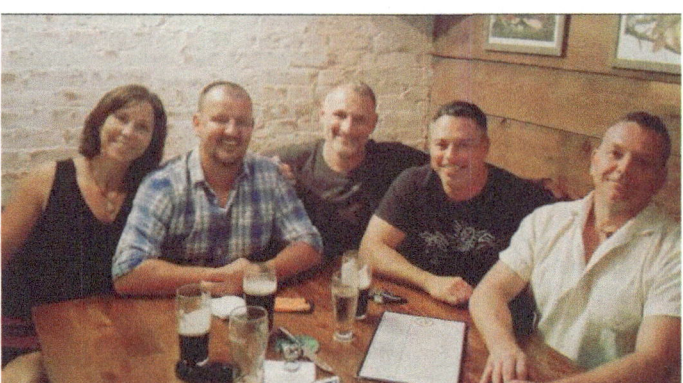

Left to right: Rachel Cosgrove, Alwyn Cosgrove, myself, Spencer Marcus and Steve Didio

What few people know about Alwyn is that he is a cancer survivor. Cancer doesn't discriminate and the timing is never good. When he was diagnosed with cancer, he had just opened a gym in California and had a huge personal following. So with his diagnosis and focus shifting to fighting for his life, he was forced to become more efficient at running his business while preparing to battle the brutal effects of chemotherapy. Basically, he had to find a way to remove himself from the day to day operations. His absence due to illness created many challenges for his gym and there was concern that without his hands-on presence, the business would fail. Alwyn realized he had to train his staff differently in order for them to share his programs with their clients. He had to enable hundreds of people to have access to his information even when he wasn't accessible. So what was the result of Alwyn training his staff to use his training programs? Alwyn's business actually grew in his absence, because his staff was able to follow his programming. While his presence was missed, his signature training styles were still being provided to his gym members and people were getting results.

Thankfully, Alwyn is healthy and still in full remission. His business in California and abroad are doing extremely well. Yet even with his busy schedule, he always makes himself available to offer his knowledge and share his expertise with a friend. Loyalty runs deep with him.

Not for Profit Influences
Lastly, I am grateful to the amazing people who've influenced and impacted my focus and desire to help my "community". I'm fortunate enough to be friends and peers with several executive directors and/or founders of some amazing not for profit organizations. In particular, I've been greatly impacted by The Avielle Foundation, Ben's Lighthouse, Dylan's Wings of Change, and Ben's Bells Project. While their missions may differ, each organization has devoted itself to helping their community in meaningful and impactful ways. What is especially inspiring to me is that each organization was born out of experiencing great personal pain and loss, and yet they were able to focus and harness their pain in order to help others. Universally these organizations help their communities by offering programs that are inclusive, educational and contribute to building healthier and more connected communities. These organizations have taught me that **compassion, love, resilience, vulnerability, and kindness are the bedrocks of a healthy community.**

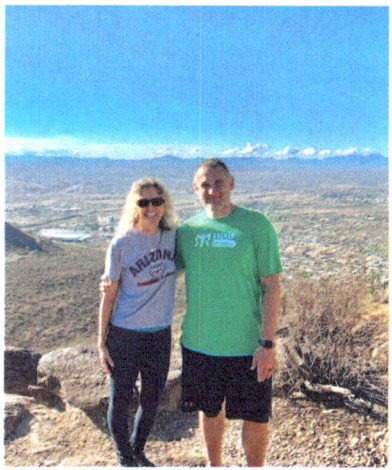

Jeannette Maré, Chief Kindness Officer and Founder of Ben's Bells Project, and myself.

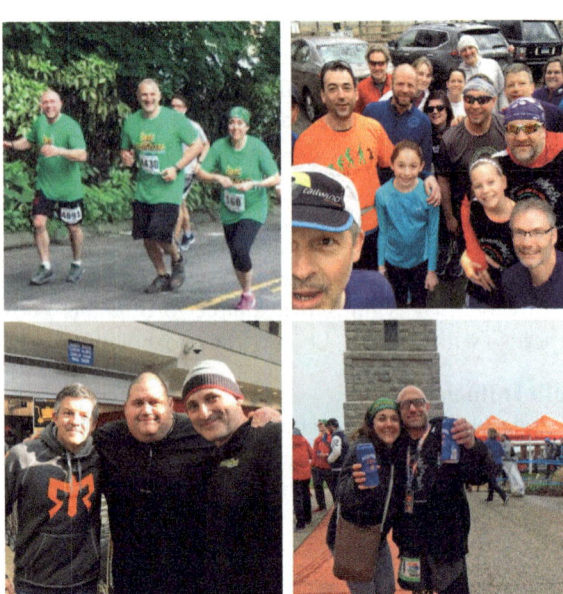

Top right: Ian Hockley and his tribe. Top left: Francine Wheeler (Ben's Lighthouse) and Jeremy Richman running a ½ marathon. Bottom right: Jeremy and Francine after completing Ragnar. Bottom left: Ian, myself and Rulon Gardner.

I also want to acknowledge the Life is Good Kids Foundation and Steve Gross. Steve is one of the most impactful speakers I've been fortunate enough to listen to. Steve has taught me and countless others about **the power of optimism** and why it is vital for children and healthy communities.

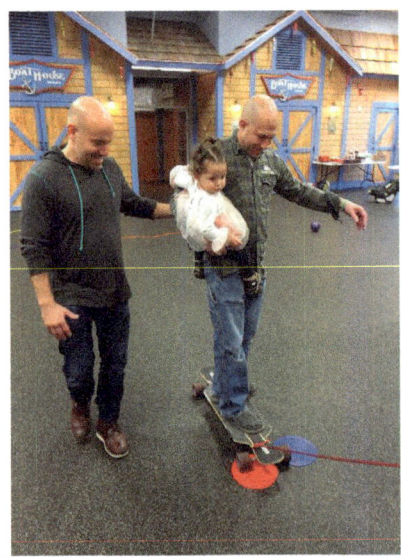

Steve Gross, Jeremy Richman and Jer's daughter in 2016.

In conclusion, The Method is a tried and proven wellness program developed from years of first-hand experience with the backing of science. However, a major component of the philosophy and methodology of The Method is about the power of human connection and its role in your fitness journey. I'm thankful to have had so many amazing leaders in my life and inspirations in the nonprofit space that impacted and helped me to connect **The Human Connection to the Science of Fitness** to truly create this program. It's because of these people that The Method is a transformational process that represents so much more than just a tool to help people lose weight and get in better shape.

Chapter 2:
Why People are Failing at Fitness

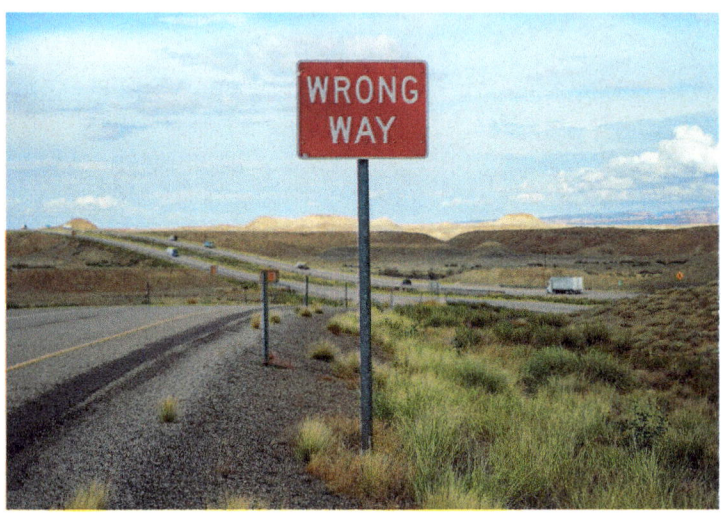

"Stop the Insanity"
What a complex challenge getting in shape is! We all know we should eat a little better and exercise a little more, but if it were that easy, we wouldn't have the obesity epidemic that this country is facing.

Have you had that moment when you see a picture of yourself, and a sinking sense of disbelief comes over you? Do you feel like you are looking at someone else? Your eyes fixate on a part of your body that appears different, worse than you remember it. Suddenly you're wondering where did you go? Maybe the moment that it hit you was a comment someone made, maybe your jeans don't fit anymore or maybe you simply don't like the way you look in the mirror? If so, join the club! As human beings, we are already predisposed to being super critical of ourselves. This coupled with society's expectations of what we should look like doesn't help.

People often make excuses or associate blame, but at some point denial shifts to acceptance, and the reality check hits! Whatever our plan has been up until now, it's not working. Often, acceptance is the first step. However, the key to a commitment to change is arming yourself with the right information and plan to allow for success. And if you really want to succeed, you have to approach this differently than you had in the past. You need to develop a successful wellness lifestyle, accept that true success won't happen overnight, and setbacks are part of the process. Failure is such a common aspect of health and fitness and it's impossible not to experience it at some point. When you think about it, every time you choose something to eat, you have the potential to fail. However, what's more important is how we respond to setbacks and how our program adapts to help us overcome obstacles and setbacks.

Eating healthy isn't always easy and is challenging for even the most disciplined athletes. What I encourage you to remember is that your slip-ups don't define you. You are not the sum of your mistakes; rather they have allowed you to become the person you are today. The past is the past, leave it there.

Many of us get down on ourselves when we overeat or make the wrong food choices. Being healthy is a lifestyle; it isn't a quick fix diet. You're going to slip up and that's okay. Forgive yourself. Love yourself. You only have one body, so my advice is that you need to learn to love it. You deserve it!

So why is it so hard to get in better shape and maintain it? The answer often lies in a faulty plan and utilizing the wrong information. Consequently, regardless of the efforts of the individual, failure is often unavoidable. So let's look at some of the common problems associated with failed fitness programs.

I had a client that came to me after experiencing some physical setbacks and weight gain while participating in a very active lifestyle. She loved going to the gym and was an active runner. Yet as she reached her mid 30's she began to slowly gain weight and her body began to break down from overuse injuries. Her determination and effort were outstanding, but her training program was flawed and was leading to failure. So what was the problem? For starters, nobody ever explained to her that excessive cardio training without strength training can lead to weight gain. She had no idea her training plan was reducing her resting metabolism and sabotaging her results. Additionally, no one ever suggested that she should have her thyroid checked as indeed she suffered from hypothyroidism, a condition which also leads to reduced metabolism and is fairly common among women. Complicating matters even further, her instinctive response to countering her weight gain by working harder was leading to more problems. As she increased her running to compensate for the weight gain, she began to develop some overuse injuries at her knees, setting off another obstacle and further sabotaging her goals. Sadly, what she needed to do from the very beginning was to create a plan that would have allowed her to **work smarter not harder.**

My client is a perfect example of the wrong information and the inability to change behavior, leading to failure. Clearly, she was motivated, as you can't run 10 miles on the weekends and be classified as lazy or unmotivated. Fortunately, after working with her for a few weeks we were able to reduce the pain in her joints by choosing better exercises and reducing overuse patterns. We were also able to create successful body fat loss strategies that helped her reach her goals. The initial weeks were tough as she fought years of misguided habits and a poor fitness strategy. Today she is stronger, more fit, and in the best shape of her life. The key was a better plan.

Let's look more closely at some of the issues that prevent us from achieving our fitness goals:

Bad information coming from the wrong people. Interestingly enough, as obesity continues to skyrocket in this country, the weight loss industry continually sells millions of dollars in books, workouts, and supplemental products. The irony is palpable and it's frustrating to see how the demand for people wanting information to change is being met with inaccuracies and half-truths. Unfortunately, this industry is selling a lot of junk and praying on people's vulnerabilities. The bottom line is that experts are not always providing a well-rounded, customizable approach to wellness. They seem to be selling one-dimensional approaches and, in my opinion, fail to provide the full wellness approach necessary for sustainable results. Visually stimulating book covers and sexy models with big smiles selling "Fun", "Easy", "Fast" fall short on delivering results.

I also caution people to be wary of trainers who are measured less on their academic background, but more by their association with celebrities or even worse, their own physical assets. Image, personality, and looks shouldn't qualify someone as an expert on health and nutrition.

Lastly, the doctors, professors, and nutritionists that represent the clinical research community are vital for the information they provide all of us. However, clinical and research knowledge without any practical or first-hand experience in how to apply the information or properly coach the movement is ineffective. In other words, while science is the basis for all information, health practitioners that have never engaged in the activity they are recommending can create a disconnect if they have no first-hand experience. There is something to be said for being on the front lines, which sometimes I'm not sure our medical community fully understands. I greatly respect and appreciate all opinions, but **wellness is a combination of science and application.** Combine those with experience and you have the best opportunity for success. Most current experts seem qualified in one, but not all these areas.

Not understanding that motivation alone doesn't equal success. I've heard countless times that people lack motivation, and that's why they are overweight! We live in a harsh society where people can make assumptions about someone based on their physical appearance. This idea that you are lazy or lack motivation if you are overweight is a cruel, shaming stigma. Suggesting someone is failing at fitness because they lack motivation oversimplifies a complicated issue and can make someone struggling with their fitness feel even worse about an already sensitive issue. Trust me, anyone that struggles with their fitness is aware when they are failing. Also, I have never met anyone that doesn't have at least some motivation to look and feel better. Whether it's for their family, their health, their self-esteem, work, etc. ... Everyone wants to feel better about how they look. I've known people that have a great work ethic, are highly motivated and successful in many areas of their lives but have failed at fitness.

We know that obesity is both genetic and environmental. Many children are classified as obese before their 10th birthday and somehow suggesting this is the result of a lack of motivation doesn't sound right.

As a society, we need to take an approach other than identifying those that fail at fitness as lazy or unmotivated. It **leads to pervasive thinking that fitness success is purely a mental discipline**. All we are doing is driving those that struggle further away. We're increasing the gap between those struggling to get in better shape and those that just can't relate because fitness or sports has always been a part of their life. Health and wellness should be an inclusive right and shaming folks doesn't create a very warm invite.

Not understanding the importance of metabolism, or more importantly, knowing how to increase it. The science is very clear on this one. Without generating, or at least preserving our lean body mass, our metabolism will decrease as we age and consequently, we will gain weight. **One of the most effective ways to increase your metabolism is to increase your lean body mass through strength training**. However, a poorly designed strength program due to a lack of understanding of the science of strength training will lead to ineffective results, injury, burnout, boredom, or disengagement altogether.

Not understanding the importance of choosing the right type of cardiovascular program. Remember the story about my client that was running excessively? Sadly, she, like so many people, never learned that the type of cardiovascular training, the intensity, the duration, and the mode of activity are crucial to creating benefits that support increasing metabolism versus breaking it down. **Cardiovascular training has multiple factors that have very specific effects on your body.** Learning how to manipulate the science of this is what makes the difference between results and frustrating failures.

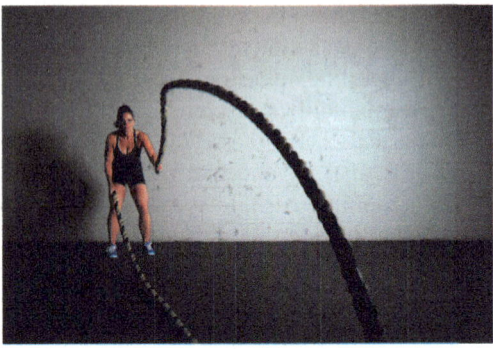

Proper Nutrition. If you thought people were confused about what exercises to do, nutrition takes that confusion to a whole new level! Let's face it, a lot of energetic fitness enthusiasts and health experts have been flooding the market with confusing and contradictory information about diet over the past 40 years. And it's not just those zany infomercials. I remember in the 80's when the USDA provided these really cool pyramid food charts.

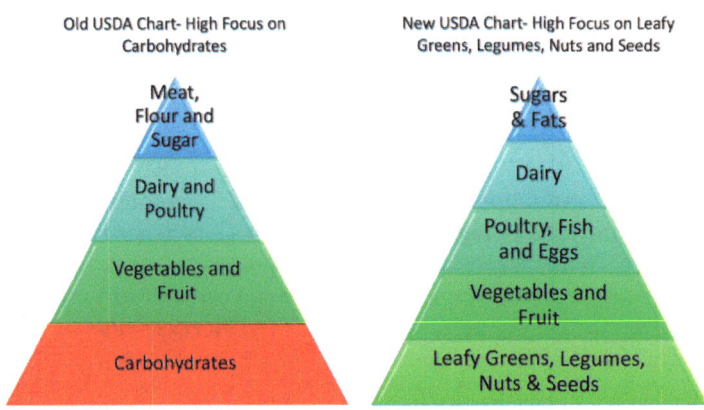

They were hung up in schools, cafeterias, taught in health class, etc. Little did we realize that these charts placed too high of an emphasis on carbohydrates. The charts also failed to differentiate between processed and unprocessed carbohydrates. People weren't being told that a processed carbohydrate doesn't resemble a natural complex carbohydrate on a molecular and nutritional level. In other words,

Wonder Bread and rice crackers aren't great representatives of the grains group. We were warned of the dangers of fat and encouraged to eat protein but the take-home was "low fat diets with plenty of carbohydrates". The low-fat campaign began and whether it was sugar-free soda or fat-free muffins, we began substituting sugar and artificial sweeteners for fat. This period is often associated with the true launch of our obesity problem. It's so ironic that the strategy to reduce weight had the exact opposite effect. Consuming fat became public enemy #1, yet somehow sugar got a pass. I remember one infomercial in particular with one of the more popular nutritional programs entitled "Stop the insanity!" The message was that you can't get fat if you don't eat fat. Eat as many potatoes as possible! As long as you avoided fat you would lose weight! Huh?

Then came the 90's and the craze became the no-carb diet. Vegetables and especially fruits became bad things. Bodybuilders preached nothing but protein and suddenly we were being told to do the exact opposite of what was recommended just a few years before. If you were keeping track, first it was Wonder Bread and potatoes then it was no fruit! I can't stomach going into the juicers, elixirs, cabbage diets, and celebrity diets, etc., it's just too frustrating and a waste of time.

So, what is the right information? The truth is that while we slipped up in the '80s with the counter fat movement, most nutritionists have been preaching accurate information this whole time. However, most people aren't interested in boring information, we want the shortcut. Basically, **eating a balanced, healthy representation of whole foods, lean proteins, fruits, and vegetables is the perfect diet**. I will discuss nutrition in detail later, but the point I'm trying to make is that everyone seems interested in the trendy, exotic diet that some movie star claims is the next miracle and it just doesn't work. Diets don't work!

Not putting "you" first. Above everything else, I think the biggest issue people face is that they don't invest in themselves like they do other facets of their lives. And people rarely prioritize themselves in the same way they would for their children or loved one's. We pay for doctors, lawyers, accountants, mechanics, etc. with the understanding that these professionals provide us with the information and plan necessary to address areas where we aren't experts. However, with fitness, people rarely invest in professionals to guide them. Combine that with this noble sense of sacrifice and selflessness that so many people adopt when they become parents or when building a career or business and suddenly you create an environment where the likelihood of succeeding at reaching your fitness levels in greatly compromised. But if you truly want to live a healthy balanced life, I believe you have to invest both time and resources to achieve this.

I recently sat down with a mentor and inspiration of mine, Jeannette Maré, who offered insight into why it's so important to make time for yourself. Jeannette speaks to the importance of self-kindness and developing strategies to reduce self-critical thinking. Her message is both inspirational and informative and her work has greatly impacted not only me, but hundreds of thousands of people. In 2002, Jeannette started a national not-for-profit organization called Ben's Bells Project. This organization is grounded in the science of kindness and its mission is "to teach individuals and communities about the positive impacts of intentional kindness and to inspire people to practice kindness as a way of life". Over the past 20 years, Jeannette has established herself as a renowned public speaker who has reshaped how people view kindness. When she and I discussed how wellness and kindness connect, she explained that focusing on your own health and wellness benefits you and others. You will be able to maintain stronger relationships with those you love when you yourself are healthier. According to Jeannette, it's not selfish to invest in your wellness. She believes your health is worth the time and cost you may invest in food, equipment, access to information, etc., because your relationships with others depend on your self-kindness.

Below are some of Jeannette's insights in her own words…

Where do you place yourself on your kindness priority list? If you're like many, it's easier for you to focus your kindness on others than on yourself.

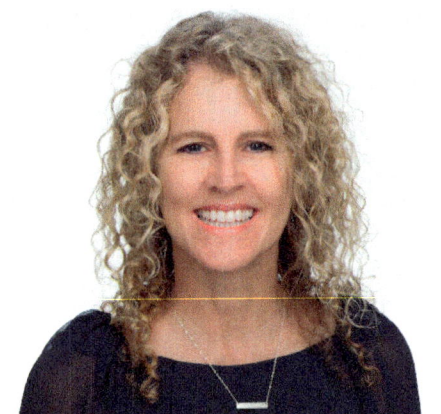

Jeannette Maré, Chief Kindness Officer and Founder of Ben's Bells Project.

You may even believe that treating yourself with kindness is selfish and that putting others first is more virtuous. The great news is that you don't have to choose between benefit for others and benefit for yourself.

Being kind to yourself is good for you AND for others and being kind to others is good for you AND for them.

That's the amazing thing about kindness and the reason I advocate putting kindness to yourself at the top of your priority list. If you treat yourself well, you will be more healthy and more emotionally fit to engage with kindness in the world. If you do not prioritize your health and wellness, you will not be fit to engage with the same level of physical, emotional, and cognitive energy.

Being kind to yourself comes in many forms but it starts with taking care of your physical self through eating well, moving your body (a lot), and getting good sleep, as is detailed in this book. From that foundation, other self-kindness and other-kindness practices that require complex emotion-regulation or cognition are more doable. Personally, my desire to be a kind and productive member of my community motivates me to be kind to myself by prioritizing my physical health. ***I can give so much more when I first give to myself.***

For more information on Ben's Bells Project, please visit www.bensbells.org.

In the upcoming chapters, we will provide accurate information to provide the structure and options to allow you to find success in wellness. As we move forward in building the foundation for this program it's important to learn from our past mistakes and hopefully this chapter has shed some light on the reasons so many of us have struggled or failed in the past. Let's remember to be kind to ourselves and let science guide us away from the pitfalls but toward the habits, exercises and nutrition needed to live our best life!

Chapter 3:
Resting Metabolic Rate (RMR)

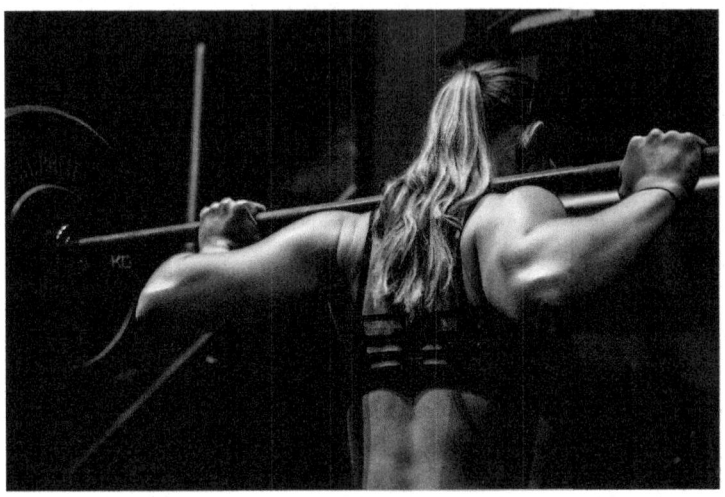

"The Fountain of Youth"
A key component of The Method and common theme throughout this book is learning how to work smarter, not harder to improve your fitness. The best way to do this is by improving your metabolism, resulting in your body burning more calories at rest. Basically, metabolism is the process in which you provide your body energy by breaking down the food you consume and combining that with oxygen. This is a fascinating and involved process, but what's relevant for us to understand is that metabolism uses a high level of calories every day. So if you can find ways to make this system more effective at burning calories, you will greatly impact your fitness. Metabolism isn't only active during exercise, it is responsible for fueling homeostasis or the body keeping a constant internal temperature and every basic function we need for survival: breathing, the heart pumping, release of hormones, blood circulation, digestion, temperature regulation, etc. Your metabolism is active every day, so taking advantage of this system is no different than earning interest on your money in a savings account. Manipulating your metabolism is like resetting your biological clock to being a teenager again. Remember when your body used to burn calories simply because it was busy building and growing your body? In upcoming chapters, we will discuss in-depth strategies to successfully develop your **Resting Metabolic Rate (RMR)** or the total number of calories burned when your body is completely at rest. We will also guide you through

strategies to avoid the vicious yo-yo effects experienced by programs that decrease your RMR.

Before we look at how to alter and improve your RMR, we first need to look at some of the inherent factors that impact your fitness capacity that cannot be altered.

Genetics: Inevitably most of us will inherit our parent's body types. In fact, Children with two obese parents are 80% more likely to be obese. We need to set fair expectations of what we want our bodies to look like and comparing yourself to an airbrushed model vs looking at your family photos is unrealistic. I'm not saying that you can't strive to look and feel better than your genetic pool, but let's start with realistic expectations and build upon that as a starting place.

Body Type: We all inherit certain body types, which are classified as ectomorphs, mesomorphs, or endomorphs. Certain body types have characteristics much more susceptible to being heavier than others. The endomorph, for example, is a person shorter in stature and more pear-shaped. This genetic body type is very susceptible to gaining weight. The ectomorph is usually taller and thinner and weight gain isn't as much of an issue. Mesomorphs fall in between the ectomorph and endomorphs. Understanding your classification and what traits are associated with that body type will help manage expectations. Regardless of your body type, your total body size will also affect your metabolism. Simply stated, the larger your total size, the higher your metabolism will be. Additionally, gender plays a role in metabolism as men will typically have higher levels of lean body mass than women.

Age Factors: By age 16.5, your fat cell amount is determined. At this point, fat cells can only expand or shrink. Obese people have much higher levels of fat cells making them more susceptible to fat storage. It is possible to increase fat cells after 16, but normally this will only happen during substantial weight gain. This doesn't mean that your fitness life is predetermined by your teenage years, but it does mean that you will have to work harder than others if you have always struggled with your weight. Also, we naturally lose muscle as we age, and consequently, our metabolism slows. Unless we engage in lean body mass generating activities, like strength training, we'll face the reality that maintaining our weight becomes more and more difficult.

Understanding some of the inherent factors listed above may be helpful to appreciate some obstacles you may face. However, what's great about metabolism is that there are several ways to manipulate your metabolism to make it work better for you. Simply said, the foods you eat and the exercises you choose have a tremendous impact on your metabolism.

3 Ways to Increase Metabolism

To succeed in increasing your metabolism, you need to understand how to develop and preserve your lean body mass. As you stoke that fire, your body will burn more calories at rest and your body fat will drop.

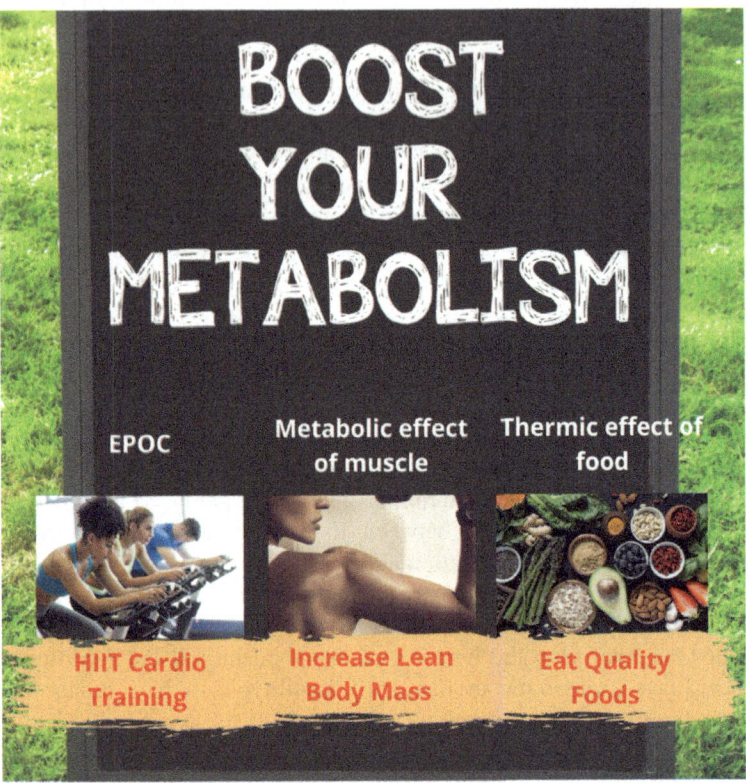

1. **Choosing the right types of cardiovascular training will preserve lean body mass and continue to burn calories after you have completed your exercise.** This specific form of cardiovascular training is called High-Intensity Interval Training or HIIT.

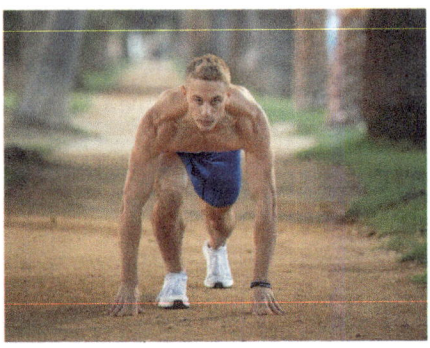

2. **Unless significant measures are taken, muscle will naturally decline.** Muscle mass decreases approximately 3-8% per decade after the age of 30. After the age of 60, this rate of decline is even higher. This can be devastating to the body as lean body mass contributes significantly to your resting metabolic rate. Knowing this is crucial to understanding why everyone needs to strength train. **Strength training is the most effective way we have to mitigate and reverse the effects of a naturally declining lean body mass.**

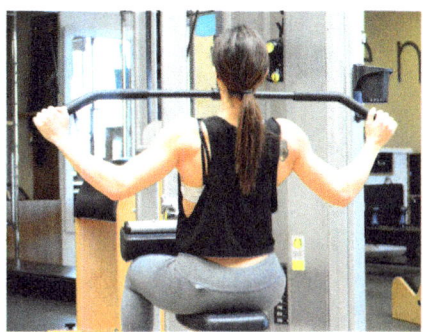

3. **Nothing is more harmful to your metabolism than depriving the body of calories or fasting.** The problem with fasting is that if you deprive your body of calories, it will act as though you are starving and burn muscle and fat as energy sources and guess what... decrease your lean body mass. So for the countless folks that have cleansed only to experience a weight spike several weeks later, you have experienced the consequence of losing valuable lean body mass. Conversely, if you learn to eat the right types of food, you will not only fuel your body with energy but will increase your metabolism.

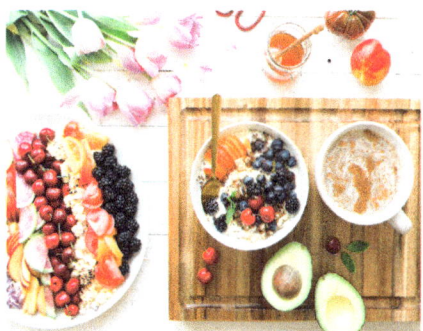

Chapters 4, 5, and 6 will provide an abundance of information on how to specifically impact your metabolism through cardiovascular training, strength training, and nutrition.

Chapter 4:
Cardiovascular Training

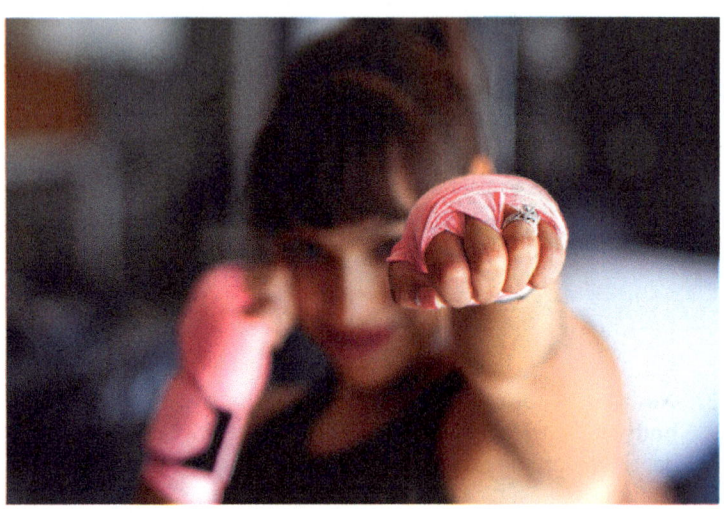

"Work Smarter, Not Longer"
There is probably more confusion regarding cardio training than any other area of wellness. Should you walk for an hour? Should you take a spin class? Maybe you heard the elliptical is the best way to lose weight? Which is better? How do different cardio training systems impact your body? People are often shocked when they learn that traditional methods of cardiovascular training could be what is undermining their weight loss efforts. Just think about it, what if your current cardio program might be the reason that you are **not** seeing results? Not your effort, will nor desire, but your plan!

Worse than the confusion that is out there is the typical thinking most people have when they decide to get themselves in better shape. What do they turn to? The throwback workout! We discussed this earlier but we've all been there, it usually starts with dusting off the New Balances, creating a good music mix, and off you go. So while visions of your former success may fill your head, unfortunately, the rules of training are much different for us than they were in our teens or early twenties. Not to mention that nothing derails a workout plan like an injury. Now, I don't want to discourage enthusiasm and the bottom line is that any activity that doesn't lead to injury is positive. However, there is a science to making the body work efficiently and effectively and as discussed earlier, effort alone doesn't equal success. So let's look at the science and begin to remove the emotion, tradition, and myths that come hand in hand with cardiovascular training.

First of all, the greatest cardio workout based on calories burned is what your body does throughout the day. No workout will match the energy expenditure required to provide the basic functions of work, rest, play, and sleep that occur on a daily basis. Let's create an optimal example and evaluate our overall activity levels separate from the 60 minutes we spend in the gym. Out of a possible 98 (guesstimate) waking hours per week, how many hours are you spending in an active state? A grueling workout 4 times a week followed by a sedentary lifestyle does not qualify as participating in a full wellness lifestyle. Sedentary jobs, TV's, computers, etc. don't require a lot of calories. You need to make a conscious effort to add a little extra physical activity to your day. Taking the stairs versus an elevator, choosing a further parking spot, yard work, etc. These simple gestures really are important and can make a world of difference. Remember we are looking for a collective strategy versus an "all or nothing" approach.

In addition to simple lifestyle changes, there are two categories of cardiovascular training to further enhance your wellness plan:

1. **High-Intensity Interval Training- HIIT:** These are exercises that incorporate short duration, high-intensity bouts of movement with mixed variables of rest, work, and intensity. Examples include boxing, spin class, sprinting, basketball, soccer etc.

2. **Low-Intensity Steady-State Training- LISS:** These exercises are long duration, low-intensity movements with consistent tempo and intensity. Examples include walking and jogging.

Now that we have our two categories, which is the best type of cardio training to get results? I have struggled with educating the traditional cardio folks more than any group. Even those that are willing to listen to science can still struggle mightily when trying to change patterns, behaviors, perceptions, and expectations.

Sometimes a picture can tell the best story. In the late '90s, a lot of articles began to feature striking pictures of world-class marathon runners and world-class sprinters. These side-by-side comparisons displayed a drastic difference in body types and most people identified the sprinter body as more desirable than the marathon runner. What's interesting is that both athletes compete at running and neither present with high levels of body fat, if any at all. When was the last time you saw an overweight world-class runner of any type? Any world-class athlete has good genetics and collegiate, professional, and Olympic athletes have all the necessary training and nutrition information available. So what explains the difference in body types? The next logical step is to look at how exactly these athletes train. Therein lies the reason for their physiques as their bodies are reflective of their training, which is drastically different.

Sprinters perform HIIT types of cardio training when they sprint. Rather than steady-state long-distance running, they focus primarily on advanced plyometrics, strength training and of course, sprinting. Marathon runners ultimately rely on long-duration cardio training. While distance runners have started to incorporate more strength training, its typically significantly less than compared to sprinters. If a world-class marathon runner looks so skinny that in some cases they even look unhealthy and their primary form of exercise is long duration cardiovascular training, we're presented with a very interesting observation. Two world-class runners with completely different body types as a result of how they train for their sport. This simple, but effective visual provides us with another example of why we should be challenging the way we think about fitness. So sprinters are validating what the experts in the fitness world have known for a while, short-duration, high-intensity bouts of energy expenditure known as HIIT to the fitness world, is the best way to burn fat and develop toned muscle.

Here are examples of why Low-Intensity Steady State Cardiovascular Training is less effective than HIIT.

Cardio training breaks down muscle, which reduces your metabolism. Every pound of muscle on your body burns roughly 6 calories a day. Breaking down your body's best way to burn calories is a critical mistake in a life of wellness. This might be your best take-home point. Don't mess with the system that is burning calories for you at rest.

Steady-state cardiovascular training rarely creates a caloric expenditure after that activity is completed. This is referred to as Energy Post Oxygen Consumption or EPOC. I will go into greater detail about this later and it should be noted that there are certain forms of HIIT that will create some form of EPOC, but the traditional slow state cardio training will not.

Cardio training can create overuse injuries due to the extensive volume of repetitions. Overuse injuries can occur in many ways, but endurance athletes and cardio-intensive fitness enthusiasts seem to lead the pack. There are so many variables that can lead to injury, but one constant predictor is flawed biomechanics or compromised joints. Think of the thousands of contacts your foot makes over a 5-mile walk or run. Now imagine faulty biomechanics repeating small irritations to a joint or muscle over and over again. It's like having a car with a flat tire and being unable to change it, but you have to drive 20 miles to work every day. Something is going to give and oftentimes it won't just be the tire. The body is the same, the knee pain (tire) will often lead to compensatory pain and consequential altered gait mechanics (how you run), ultimately breaking down other joints.

Cardio training is often very time consuming, and many times people list time restraints as one of their biggest hurdles to obtaining fitness. Also, because traditional cardiovascular training doesn't have a carryover effect (EPOC), the calories you burn in the moment are all you have. When you combine these factors, you can see why slow steady cardiovascular training can often be the least effective use of time for obtaining results. Your fitness life could be so much more effective if you choose exercises that continue to burn calories after you are done with your workout.

Low-intensity steady-state (LISS) can create a false sense of long-term accomplishment. For example, those that have been encouraged that walking as a form of exercise is enough, are being misled. While there are many physical and emotional benefits to walking, rarely does this lead to transformation. Again, I'm not discouraging walking or any movement for that matter, but we can't rely on high volume, low-intensity cardio strategies as an indefinite form of training. This type of cardio should be paired with other forms of exercise to truly contribute to an effective wellness plan.

LISS doesn't necessarily promote stronger bones or increased joint integrity. There is a positive effect on bone density with any weight-bearing activity, but the stimulation of increasing bone density from traditional cardio activities isn't nearly as effective as strength training. Meaning that for anyone looking to prevent osteoporosis, strength training is a much more effective measure.

The net calories burned during steady-state cardio training doesn't always justify the appetite increase and post-activity caloric consumption. People aren't always working as hard as they think and perceived exertion won't always balance out the actual caloric balance necessary to lose weight. This can be said for any activity, but high volume cardio is often associated with lower intensities vs HIIT.

So now that it seems that we have bashed low-intensity steady-state cardiovascular training, let's pull back a bit and acknowledge again that any movement is good and there are plenty of great qualities associated with this form of training. However, as we are trying to follow the science and provide the best information possible for successful wellness strategies, we have to objectively look at why it isn't always the best choice. With that being said, here are some of the positive qualities and why we still need to include low-intensity steady-state cardio in some capacity into our wellness plan.

Advantages of LISS cardiovascular training:
- It is an efficient way to burn acute calories.
- It helps reduce the risk of heart attack, high cholesterol, high blood pressure and diabetes.
- It increases your lung capacity.
- For many people, this is the easiest way to begin working out.
- It helps to reduce stress.
- It helps you to sleep better.

I could go on, but you get the point. We know low-intensity cardiovascular training is healthy for you, but we need you to also understand that it's often the least effective strategy to change your body.

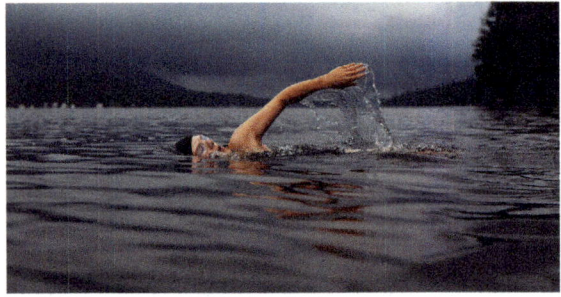

So if steady-state isn't the answer, what exactly is HIIT and why does it work? High-intensity interval training (HIIT) is the form of cardiovascular training associated with high-intensity outbursts followed by intermittent rest. HIIT training uses the anaerobic energy system which, unlike the aerobic system, doesn't require oxygen as an energy source. The absence of oxygen as an energy source allows for faster fuel sources to support explosive movements. So while energy is produced faster, the anaerobic system is far less efficient at sustaining movement compared with cardiovascular training.

Think back to the sprinter and their workouts. Fast, explosive movements with intermittent rest. Other examples of HIIT are boxing, tennis, basketball, soccer, hockey, etc. When you think of these types of activities, you might identify that they are all associated with intensity. The idea is that you perform an activity at high intensity followed by intermittent bouts of recovery. There are so many ways to program this, but conservatively you can start with a 1 to 4 work to rest ratio. You can measure this in time or distance. For example, run one lap hard then jog 4 laps for recovery. Or cycle as hard as you can for 60 seconds then pedal slowly for 4 minutes. As you progress, continue to reduce the recovery ratio, but always allow yourself to express high intensity. The outcome produced by the intensity level is ultimately what creates the training effect that translates into results.

Specifically, I'm talking about a physiological response called Energy Post Oxygen Consumption or EPOC. As mentioned above, this is an amazing response where your body must burn additional calories after your workout to assist in the recovery from performing HIIT. In other words, these are bonus calories that keep burning even after your workout. **It's estimated that an additional 6-15% of the calories you burned during a HIIT movement will be burned during EPOC recovery**. So if you burned 300 calories during a spin class, you can expect to burn an additional 18-45 calories after your workout. This response is only elicited with HIIT and some forms of intense strength training.

Another advantage to HIIT training is that it will help preserve lean body mass wherein traditional cardio training breaks down muscle and uses it for energy. As we continue to develop strategies to improve metabolism, **nothing could be more detrimental than to actually lose muscle while training.**

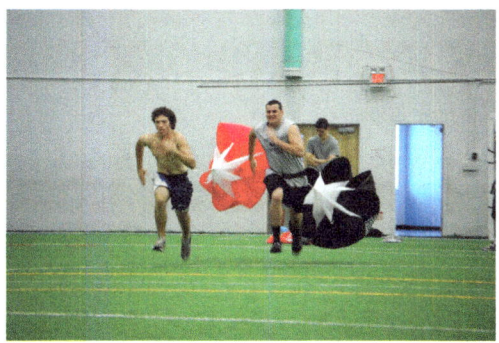
NHS football speed training.

In addition to preserving lean body mass, HIIT training activates fast-twitch fibers. Fast-twitch fibers are responsible for balance, power, coordination, etc. and are much harder to train than slow-twitch fibers. This will be discussed more in-depth during the next chapter but for now, don't think of power as only expressed or needed by high-end athletes. For example, the elderly need fast-twitch fibers to help prevent falls and improve reflexes and balance. **From the standpoint of how best to manipulate your metabolism, HIIT is the clear winner and should occupy a larger space in your wellness plan.** Remember our goal is to have your body work harder for you to get the results you want.

The benefits of HIIT include:
- Boosts your metabolism.

- Burns more calories in a shorter period of time.
- Burns calories hours after your workout.
- When combined with strength training, it will decrease fat, not muscle.
- Increases your anaerobic endurance.
- Recruits fast-twitch fibers.
- Good for heart health.

Below is a list of some of my favorite cardiovascular training options. While my choices are personal favorites, I also recommend them as they are very effective at burning calories. You can also apply HIIT training principles to any movement, so don't worry if you don't see your favorite cardiovascular activity. For example, if you want to include bike riding, include sprint intervals as part of your workout and/or choose a course with hills versus maintaining a consistent pace over a set period of time. Or, if you really want to simplify this, take a spin class, as most of these classes are designed specifically to incorporate HIIT. Also, remember that utilizing your upper body for cardiovascular activity is much more effective at burning calories, that's why I love boxing, rowing and swimming as effective cardio choices. Lastly, and maybe most important, remember to start with activities that you will enjoy.

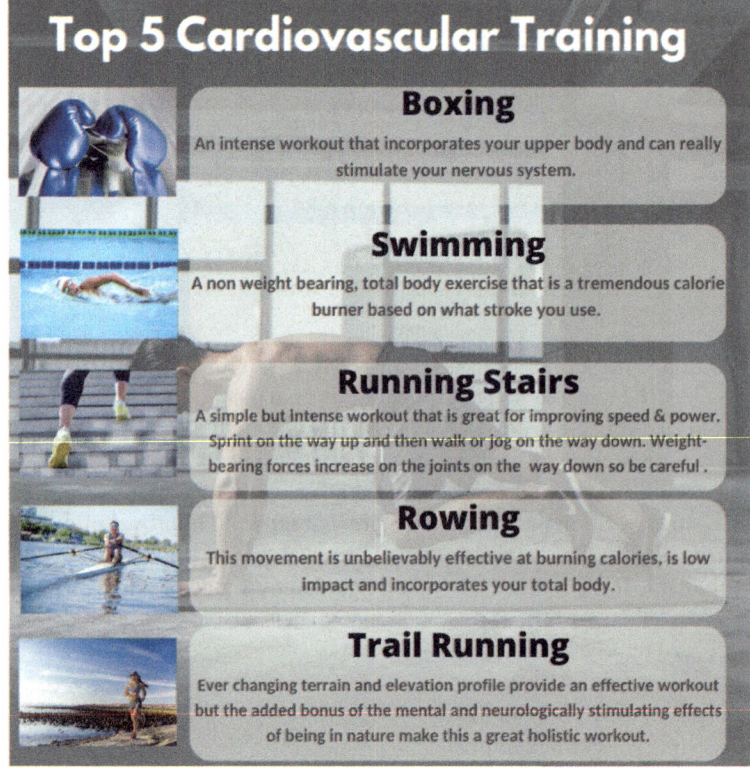

In closing, I hope I've explained the advantages of HIIT and provided you with some choices that will make cardiovascular training work better for you. I really want to emphasize that I want you to incorporate activities that you enjoy and will continue to motivate you versus only selecting what might be extreme choices for you. If you are a walker, that doesn't mean that I'm suddenly saying that you need to go to the track and do nothing but sprints. In fact, an extreme change like that can burn you out emotionally and physically. Personally, I love distance running and I incorporate it into my training even though it scientifically isn't the most effective choice. But distance running falls somewhere between therapy and a spiritual experience and this is essential to a holistic approach to wellness for me. My point is that LISS cardiovascular training can still play a significant role in the wellness spectrum. However, most people need to focus on including more HIIT cardiovascular training to achieve the results that have eluded them. Let's just make sure we transition to this approach in a healthy, effective way that will lead to lifestyle changes that are sustainable.

Chapter 5:
Strength Training

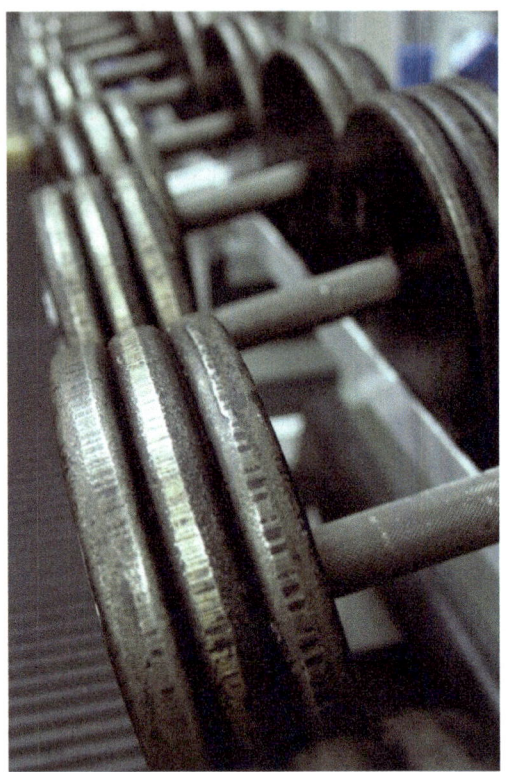

"Build the Body that will Work for You"
The goal of this book is to inform and share years of experience. However, certain topics like how to properly strength train and nutrition, are extremely in-depth with layers of content and scientific explanation that make providing slices of relevant talking points a challenge. If you are interested in learning more about any of these areas, please look at my references at the end of this book for resources.

Strength training is potentially the most important part of your wellness plan, but it is also the biggest challenge for most people to successfully implement. As referenced earlier, lean body mass drives your resting metabolism. A higher metabolism equates to more calories being burned at rest. Think of what life is like for active teenagers. As their bodies are quickly developing, they seem to eat everything in sight but not gain weight. Well, a lot of that is attributed to their active metabolism that supports their accelerated growth. But as many of us have experienced, maintaining the eating habits of our youth with a less effective metabolism quickly leads to weight gain. So let's jump-start this amazing system (metabolism), start burning more calories at rest, and recapture some of our youth.

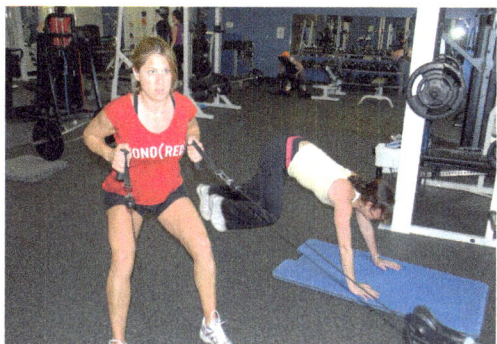

Fitness Loft training.

However, before we get too excited about how you can set the clock back and engage the "fountain of youth", we need to dig a bit deeper to understand the science of strength training.

Strength training is a form of exercise where an external load is applied to the body. When the body recruits and contracts muscle fibers to counter this external load, a specific effect takes place on the muscles involved with that movement. Based on the repetitions, speed of movement, rep count, or duration of time that the exercise is placed under tension, certain physiological responses take place in your body. Specifically, on a cellular level micro-traumas occur at the muscle, which results in your body regenerating and healing the micro-level tears, leading to increased lean body muscle. There are multiple factors that influence the outcome of strength training, and your knowledge of how to manipulate these factors is essential to achieving the desired results you want.

One key variable is the number of repetitions. Typically, the number of repetitions ranges from as little as 1 to 3 for expressions of power to as high as 15 to 20 for hypertrophy or muscle development. The low rep range suggests a heavy load is being lifted or a movement is being performed very quickly. Both have a similar neurological effect and create power. The higher rep ranges create a longer time under tension for the muscular system being affected and lead to hypertrophy or muscle building. However, exceeding too many repetitions or not creating levels of intensity where you reach failure, may not create any true strength effect. In other words, if you take a class called strength training and you do 300 bicep curls at a time, it's not strength training but muscular endurance training. Most experts will cap the repetition amount at 15 to 20 to still qualify as strength training. Another variable is measuring the duration of time that a muscle is under tension that will predict the outcome. Regardless of whether its reps or time under tension, if you exceed too many repetitions you will shift from strength to endurance, which doesn't really stimulate lean body mass growth. In other words, it's like thinking walking will strengthen your legs. While there is some general strengthening that takes place, ultimately you are conditioning versus creating the stimulus for lean body mass development.

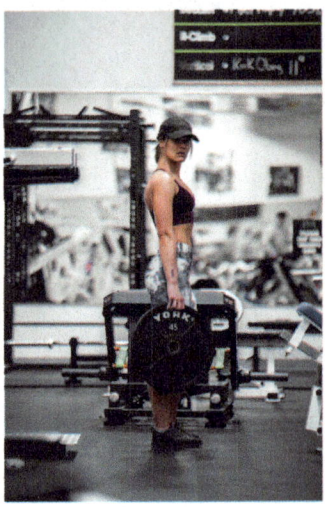

Measuring intensity is also a major variable to obtain the desired results. If you aren't applying the right intensity, you won't see the benefits. If your goal repetition count is 12, then you should be struggling as you reach your end repetitions. You should also be able to measure improvement to assess intensity. If you have been using the same weight for an exercise for several weeks, chances are your intensity levels aren't effective as you should have gotten stronger and your current weight isn't enough of a challenge. Implementing strategies to assess intensity is vital. Probably the most effective tool to measure intensity is a heart rate monitor. You can't fake a heart rate and there is no better measure to let you know how hard you are working. Technology is amazing and there are a ton of apps and devices tied to your smartphone or smartwatch to help monitor your heart rate.

Strength training's impact on changing your body is significant on multiple levels:

> ***For every new pound of muscle you build on your body, you will burn an additional 6 calories per day during rest.*** Think about it, if you gain two pounds of muscle, increase your activity, eat a little better, then "Presto!", it's a new body. The benefits don't end there.

Strength training will produce a post-exercise energy demand from the body creating a long-lasting elevated metabolism *or as was discussed earlier, energy post oxygen consumption (EPOC). Do you remember that term from HIIT? This is one of the most important concepts. EPOC addresses the energy the body has to use to restore depleted oxygen levels and cellular restoration as a result of your workout. EPOC is activated when you exert at 80% or more of your maximum heart rate.*

Strength training is also the most effective way to increase bone density. Strength training allows you to strengthen your nervous system, proprioceptive system, joints, and muscles.

It can help you improve your posture and protect you from injury because it allows you to perform specific exercises to address internal, intrinsic muscles in conjunction with large muscles.

Strength training is unbelievably adaptable with countless different types of exercises, modifications, sets, reps, load schemes, etc. The point is that a **strength program can be customized for anyone and everyone can achieve some type of benefit.** The same cannot be said for cardio training which is much less dynamic and doesn't lend itself to customization.

Where and how to start strength training. While strength training offers a wide variety of exercises to choose from, "keep it simple"! There are several movement patterns that need to be addressed to create a full-body workout. Looking at the movement type versus the actual exercise will help organize your workouts. For example, a horizontal compound press can be expressed as a bench press, push up, seated machine bench press, etc. Viewing exercises in this manner will help you both organize your workouts and provide variety and options that will both stimulate your nervous system and motivation.

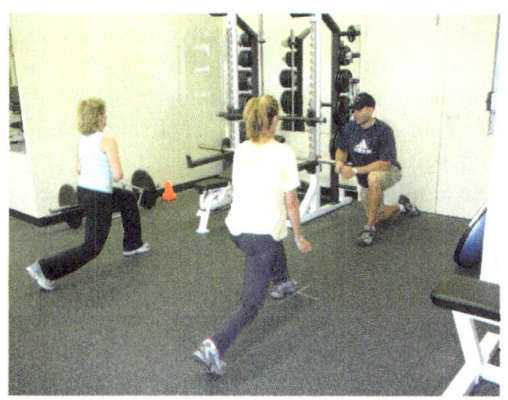

Here is a sample of how to choose movement patterns and then fill in the exercise you want. If you follow this method, you can constantly change the exercises while still performing an effective, functional workout.

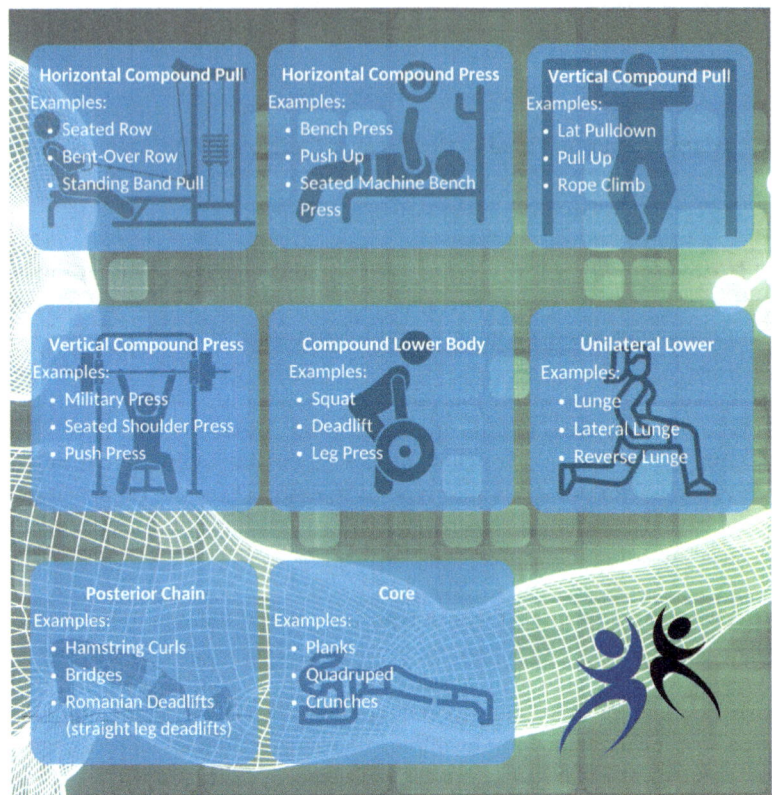

Compound Movements vs Isolation. When you think about exercise selection when strength training, think of prioritizing large muscle groups first before addressing small muscles. Specifically, **an exercise that requires at least two joints to facilitate the movement is called a compound movement. An exercise that only engages one joint is known as an isolated movement.** The logic follows that when your first few exercises (primary) are compound they will activate more muscles, creating more exertion, energy, and functionality. A common example is doing a back exercise like a pull-down (which engages your Latissimus Dorsi and elbow flexors), before doing a bicep curl (isolated). By doing the compound movement first, you can follow later with the isolated exercise effectively. However, if you pre-fatigue your biceps before doing the lat pulldown, you will decrease the efficiency of the movement. **So compound training is not only more effective, but it also mimics functional movement patterns and can translate to your body being more productive with**

activity. Think of the lat pull down again and try to visualize what that pulling motion looks like compared to just bending your elbow joint while doing a bicep curl. You will hopefully observe that we rarely use isolated joint motions in functional movement patterns.

Spot Reduction. I am often asked whether you can do exercises that will target fat reduction or "spot reduction". If you haven't heard the term spot reduction, how about the idea that doing crunches is the best way to lose the fat around your midsection? **So we are clear, this is a completely false concept that suggests performing an exercise and strengthening a particular area of the body will reduce the surrounding fat.** Fat and muscle are two absolutely different entities. Using the example of training your abdominals, if you strengthen the muscles in the midsection but do not address the fat covering them, you will create a more functional and stronger mid-section but your appearance will not alter. Body fat has no relation to the muscle activity below it. Sadly, only when your overall body fat decreases will we notice changes in those stubborn areas. I say sadly because often our trouble spots are the last areas to show the improvement we so desperately want. The only way to lose fat is through total-body strength training, proper nutrition, and correctly implemented cardio training.

What is better, Machines or Free Weights? I normally recommend training with free weights (functionally) versus machines when doing your primary exercises, but machines play a very important supplemental role with strength training. I'm a strong believer that when we strength train, we are really trying to build a body that will serve us for a lifetime. That means the movements we perform in the gym should transfer to real life. Your goal isn't to max out a selectorized (machine) leg press. Your goal is to produce leg strength that will allow you to safely and efficiently run, jump, hike, play, etc. **Strength training should address all aspects of movement including balance, coordination, flexibility, and power. So try to use fewer machines and more free weights as they will challenge your body in a more functional manner.**

Another problem with machine-based training is that due to the simplicity of the movement, oftentimes the machine exercise won't recruit the stabilization muscles and proprioceptive muscles. Stabilization and proprioceptive muscles are vital for functionality and injury prevention as their job is to protect the body from breakdown and improve its response to a loss of balance. Machines also break the pattern of the agonist-antagonist relationship. The body's muscles naturally serve as braking systems, meaning when one side recruits muscle to contract (agonist), the other side must recruit opposing muscles (antagonist) to slow down the movement. When using a machine, there is often a pulley or counterweight component that slows the movement versus the antagonist muscles that fire during free weights and real-life movement patterns.

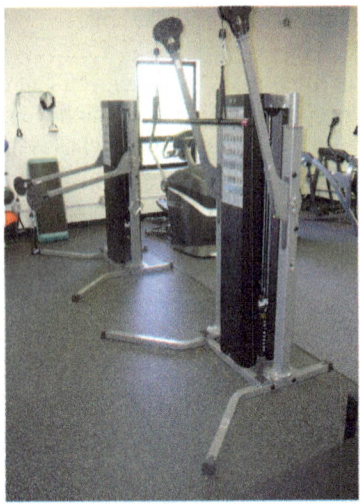

Now, before we give up on machines, remember I did say that they play an important role. When simpler movements are applied, the capacity for intensity can go up. For beginners, it might be more effective to do a machine exercise, which will be simpler to execute than a free weight movement. Machines also provide mechanical advantages to certain movements where free weights cannot. You really can't modify a bodyweight pull up unless you have someone spotting you or you are using a supportive device like a band. This creates a huge obstacle for most people in that a pull up is extremely difficult and is limited to only your body weight as the resistance. However, a selectorized lat pulldown uses the same muscles as a pull-up, but can very easily allow you to use a weight that can be performed at high repetitions. Secondarily, the lat pulldown can actually be a tool to get you better at performing a pull-up.

Strength Training Program

Now that we've gone through some of the basic principles of resistance training, I'd like to provide you with some sample workouts as well as guidance on movements you should include in your exercise routine and movements you should avoid. These basic suggestions will give you an idea of how many different ways there are to strength train, as variation and variety are great tools to achieving strength. The more diverse your exercise toolbox is and the more knowledgeable you become with program design, the better your results will be. Some of the workouts I list below will also demonstrate that you don't need a lot of equipment and it doesn't have to be expensive to workout. A major theme of this book is to provide solutions, not problems, so hopefully we are demonstrating that there is something out there for all of us, no matter what the constraint may be. With that being said, please use these suggestions to provide you with exposure to the many different options, but don't implement these workouts as a customized plan. These workouts are very generic in their suggested variables: exercise choice, set, repetition and rest. To create an effective workout plan, you would need to manipulate the variables based on your fitness level, goals and working knowledge of how to perform these movements. Also, me providing an image of an exercise isn't a substitute for learning the proper form and technique. I strongly recommend seeking guidance from a certified strength coach or personal trainer to help you safely learn each exercise.

When creating a workout plan for strength training, you need to account for 3 components of your workout:
- **The pre-workout** which consists of elevating your heart rate and preparing your body to perform the exercises designated in the workout. This can include different types of stretching and drills with a goal of decreasing injury while also increasing performance.
- **The workout** which consists of choosing the right exercises, sets, repetitions, recovery, etc. to create the desired outcome.
- **The post-workout** which will allow your body to recover from the workout by reducing your heart rate and implementing stretching to help with range of motion.

Pre-Workout Protocols

General (cardio) Warmup- Choose an activity to elevate your heart rate for at least 10 minutes. Consult with your doctor for a target heart rate, but 70% of your max heart rate is a generally suggested heart rate goal.

Optional- **Myofascial Release (Foam Roller)-** Address any tight areas with this technique before beginning exercise. The foam roller can reduce tightness by releasing trigger points that often lead to range of motion restrictions. Myofascial release is also advantages for athletes as it doesn't reduce the elastic power potential of muscle. Suggestions vary, but typically rolling over a trigger area for 20 seconds will achieve the desired result. The foam roller is an inexpensive option but there are other tools and techniques to achieve myofascial release.

Optional- **Static Stretch-** Address areas with a 20 second hold that due to tightness will impede functional range of motion. This stretch is only recommended before a workout if there is a muscle or joint that's range of motion is so restricted that it will impede your ability to safely perform a movement. Static stretching is very effective at increasing range of motion, but the process in which it does this can also decrease the stored elastic power in the muscles.

Optional- **Muscle Activation Drills-** These drills will properly fire and engage muscles that will be called upon during your exercise program. Activation drills can also be injury prevention exercises as both strengthen and activate certain muscles that often play the role of supporting larger muscles. When these smaller muscles are activated before a workout, they can enhance the effectiveness of a group of muscles working synergistically.

Highly Recommended- **Dynamic Stretch-** Are a sequence of stretches and movement's that effectively excite the body neurologically and physiologically while not sacrificing the potential power of muscles (like static stretching). These stretches require a 2 second hold and feel more like exercises in that they require balance, coordination and more exertion that the traditional stretch. These stretches are often used by athletes before practice and competition and provide a fun challenging way to get your body ready for your workout.

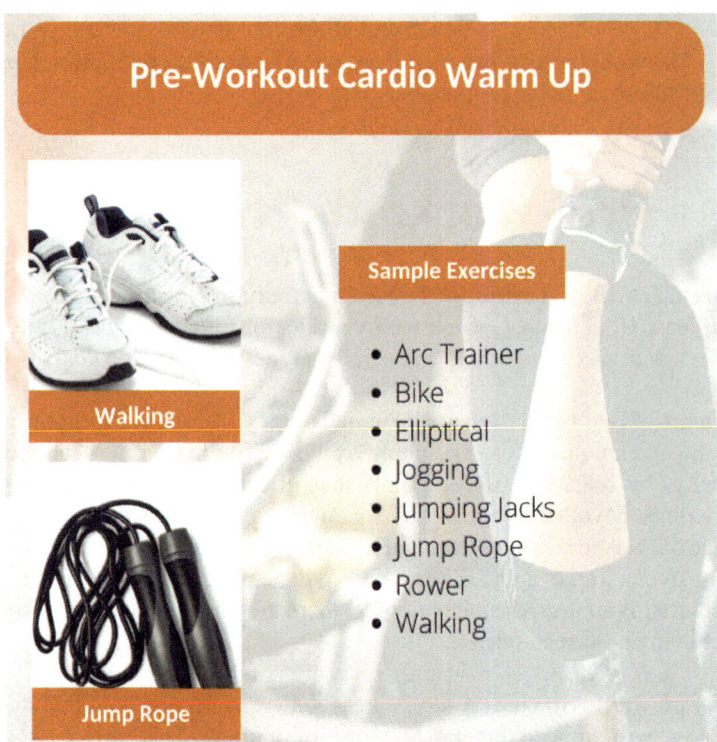

Pre-Workout Cardio Warm Up

Walking

Jump Rope

Sample Exercises

- Arc Trainer
- Bike
- Elliptical
- Jogging
- Jumping Jacks
- Jump Rope
- Rower
- Walking

Pre-Workout Myofascial Release

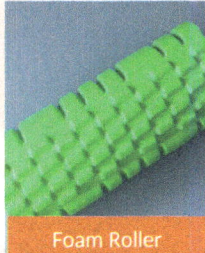
Foam Roller

Sample Tools

- Foam Roller
- Lacrosse Ball
- Massage Ball
- Massage Gun
- Massage Stick
- Trigger Point Cane/Hook

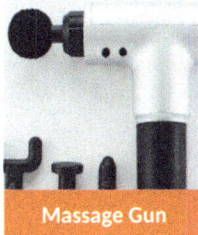
Massage Gun

Pre-Workout Static Stretch

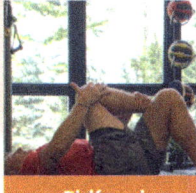
Piriformis

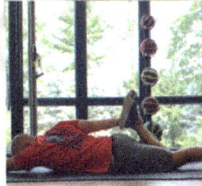
Quadruceps

Sample Stretches

Lower Body
- Adductors
- Abductors
- Gastrocnemius
- Glutes
- Hamstring
- Hip Flexors
- Soleus
- Piriformis
- Quadruceps

Upper Body
- Biceps
- Lattisimus Dorst
- Pectoralis Major
- Pectoralis Minor
- Rotator Cuff
- Tricpes

Pre-Workout Muscle Activation

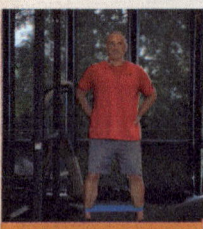
Bandwalks

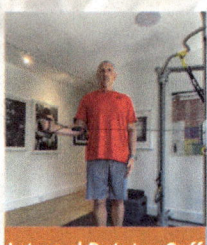
Internal Rotator Cuff

Sample Movements

- Bridges
- Bandwalks
- External Rotator Cuff
- Internal Rotator Cuff
- Hip Circles
- Hip Abduction
- Quadruped

Pre-Workout Dynamic Stretching

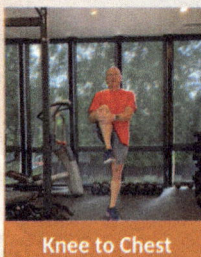
Knee to Chest

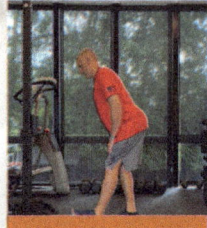
Hamstring

Sample Stretches

- Caterpillar
- Hamstring
- Knee to Chest
- Lunge Rotation
- Piriformis Cradle
- Push Up Rotation
- Quad/Calf Reach
- Scorpion
- Spiderman
- Squat Press Apart
- T Stretch

The Workout

Now that we have gone over some pre-workout suggestions, let's look at the actual exercise program design. I've outlined a basic workout for each of the following areas listed below. Based on your goals, or maybe your restrictions, find the program that looks right for you!

Program Selection Overview:

3 Day Total Body Strength Training Program- This program design allows for a challenging total body workout that requires 1-2 days of rest in between workouts. The exercise selection focuses on functional compound movements and is very effective for the individual that can only strength train 2-3 days a week.

4 Day Total Body Strength Program (quad dominant push vs posterior chain pull)- This workout design allows for back-to-back workout days. This functional four day a week program is used by athletes and folks looking to obtain aggressive results. In theory, because you are using opposing muscles each workout, potential micro tearing and soreness will be broken up more effectively.

Bodybuilder Splits- As the name implies, this program is used by bodybuilders. This workout relies on a heavy concentration of volume on certain muscles, allowing for operative aesthetic results. In other words, this workout is very effective at developing certain muscle groups. However, this approach is non-functional in nature, and therefore, is one of my least favorite program design concepts. With that being said though, this workout is a great change of pace when used sparingly and can be an effective stimulus to break up plateaus.

Supersets- Supersets fall into the HIIT (high interval intensity training) and time under tension categories as they create situations where your body is being asked to double the volume of resistance it would normally experience during strength training. With very little rest, you go from one exercise right into another one. This can be accomplished in multiple ways, but I'm providing two samples. One superset incorporates supportive muscles (agonist) where you start with a large muscle group movement and then immediately perform another exercise with a supportive, smaller muscle.

The other technique is to go from a large muscle group movement to an opposing muscle (antagonist) group exercise. Both superset techniques have distinct advantages. Supportive muscle supersets provide additional volume to smaller secondary muscles, creating greater opportunity for cellular breakdown and results. Where antagonize, or opposing muscle supersets, provide a more intense overall workout as both exercises selected are compound in nature, requiring more energy compared to an isolated supportive muscle exercise.

Power Training Upper and Lower Body- Power Training is typically reserved for more advanced lifters as either the skill set required or the weight selected increase the risk of injury. The upside is that these types of exercise programs will develop the fast twitch fibers needed to improve explosive capabilities by athletes.

Home Gym (budget)- Home gym workouts are designed to use very little equipment and still provide adequate resistance to create a great workout. The limitation of the equipment and space of your home gym are determining factors. With that being said, I've provided a workout you can do with only investing in a TRX or theracord and physio ball.

Outdoor Workout- Outdoor workouts create a great change of pace. As you move away from the confines of your gym, you'll experience the benefits of fresh air, changing terrain and the stimulation of seeing new people and having new experiences based on your location. There are limitations to the effectiveness of the workouts from a performance standpoint, but when used appropriately these workouts can reinvigorate a stale program. Similar to the home gym workout, they are also very budget friendly. Most of this equipment can be kept in a backpack, tight around the waist, or yes, stored in a stylish fanny pack.

Beginners 101- For children or adults just starting to workout, there is nothing more important than learning the right technique and how to control your own body weight before externally loading with weights or trying more advanced exercises. I'd suggest the following program as it will challenge you to master the basic movement patterns that the body will perform during strength training, while initially reducing risk.

These sample workouts don't qualify anyone to repeat the exercises listed before gaining clearance from a health care provider. I would also advise consulting with a wellness professional for the safest and most effective way to learn how to do these exercises.

Additionally, these samples are just samples. They don't thoroughly cover every aspect of your workout and more importantly they don't account for the vital information that needs to be obtained by a professional health care provider before suggesting exercises or manipulating variables for someone.

3 Day Total Body Strength Training Program

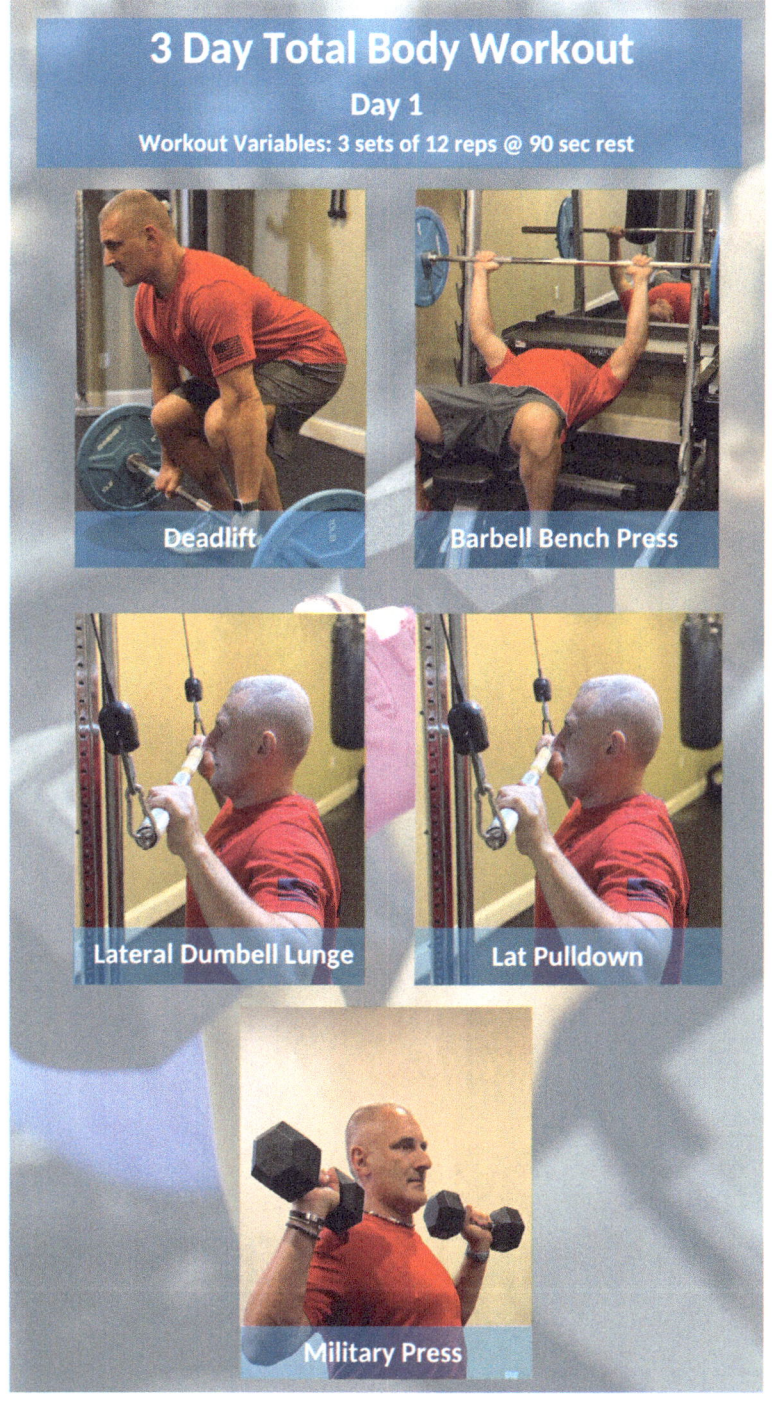

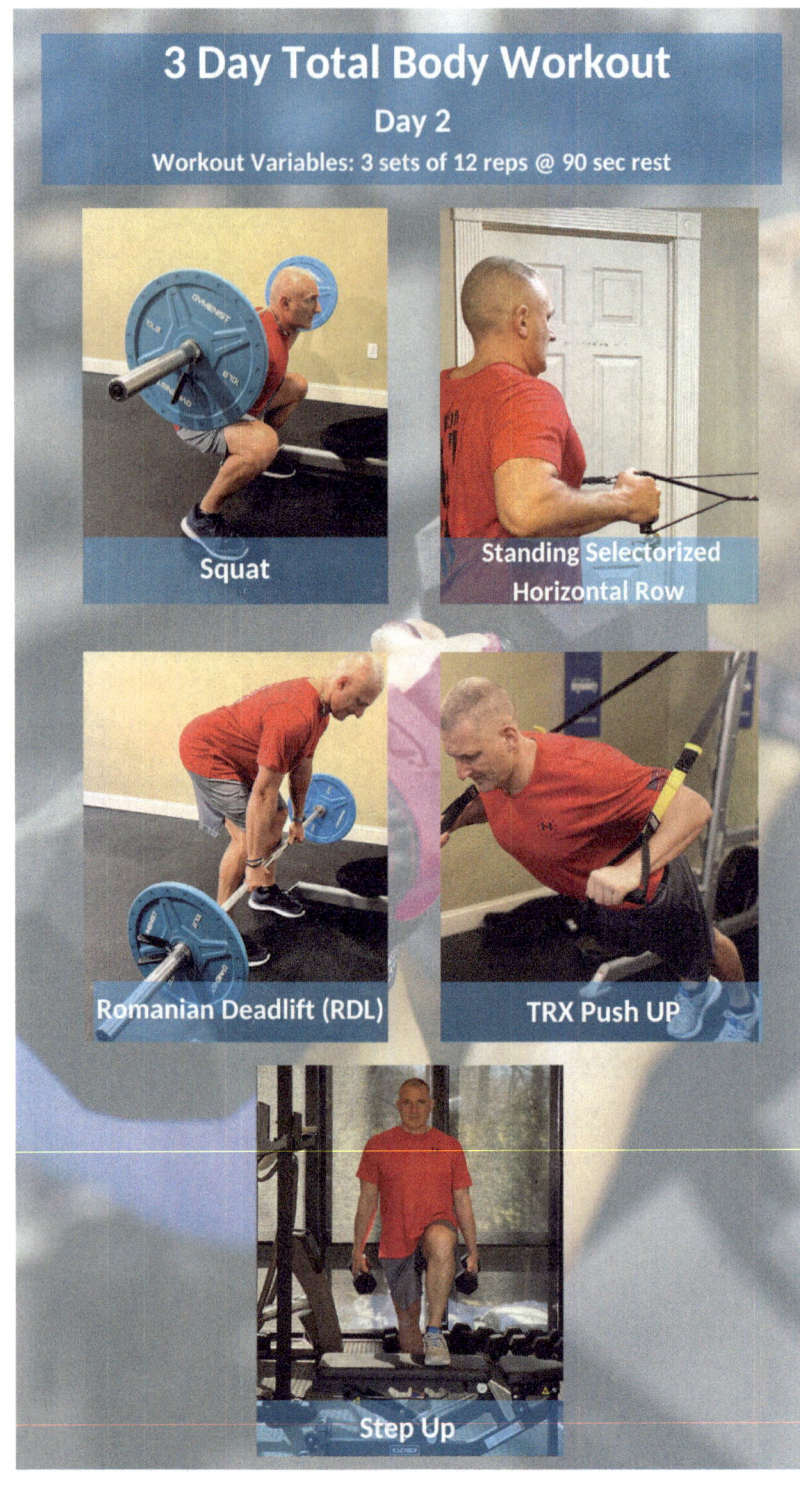

3 Day Total Body Workout
Day 3
Workout Variables: 3 sets of 12 reps @ 90 sec rest

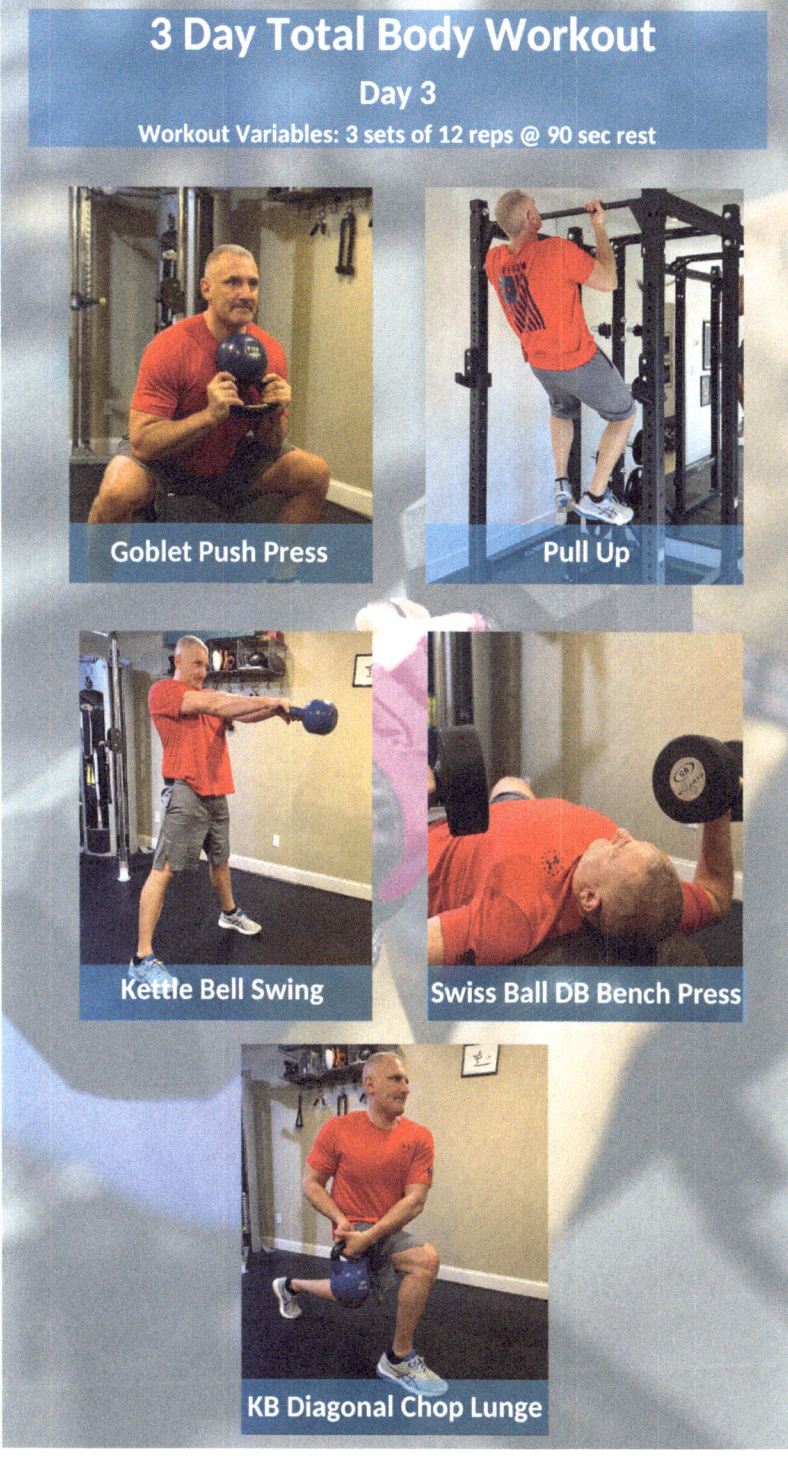

Goblet Push Press

Pull Up

Kettle Bell Swing

Swiss Ball DB Bench Press

KB Diagonal Chop Lunge

4 Day Total Body Strength Program

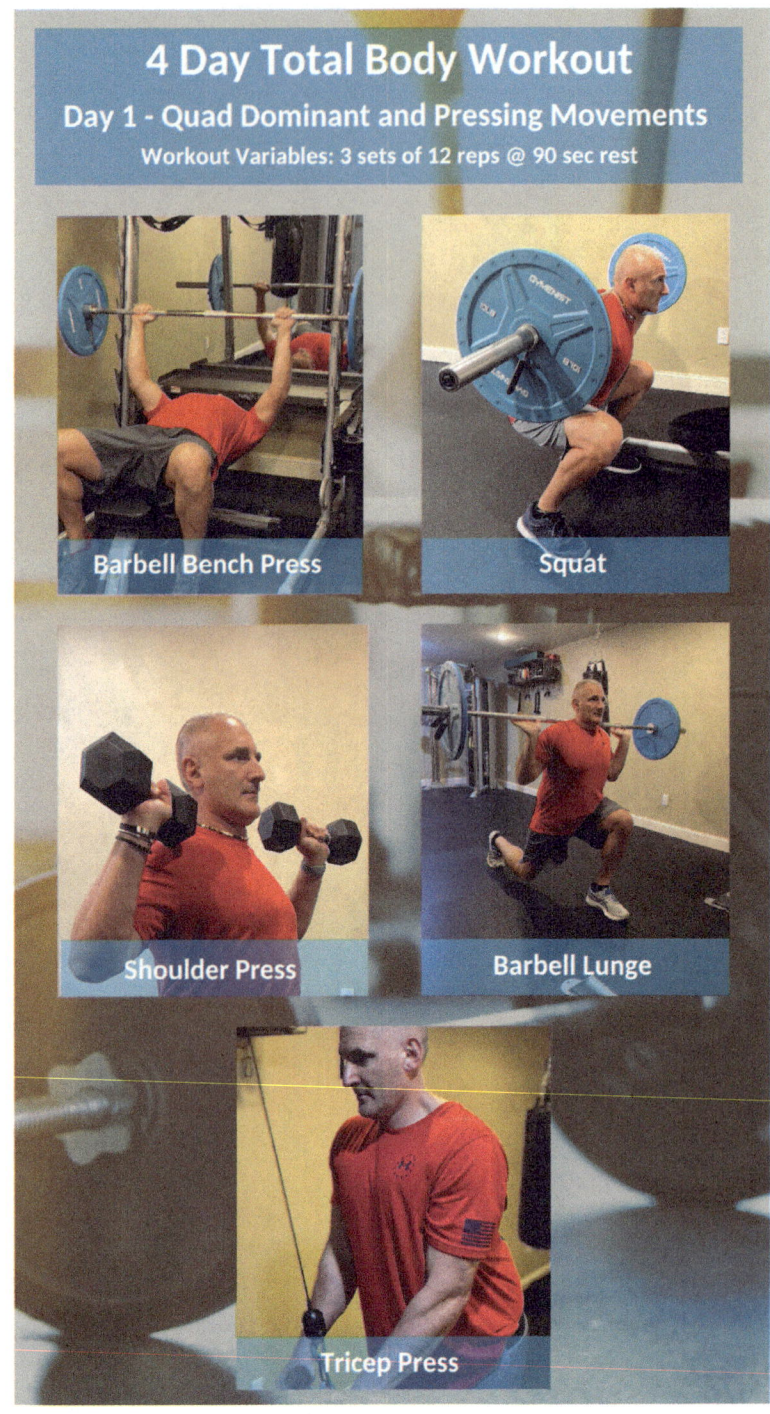

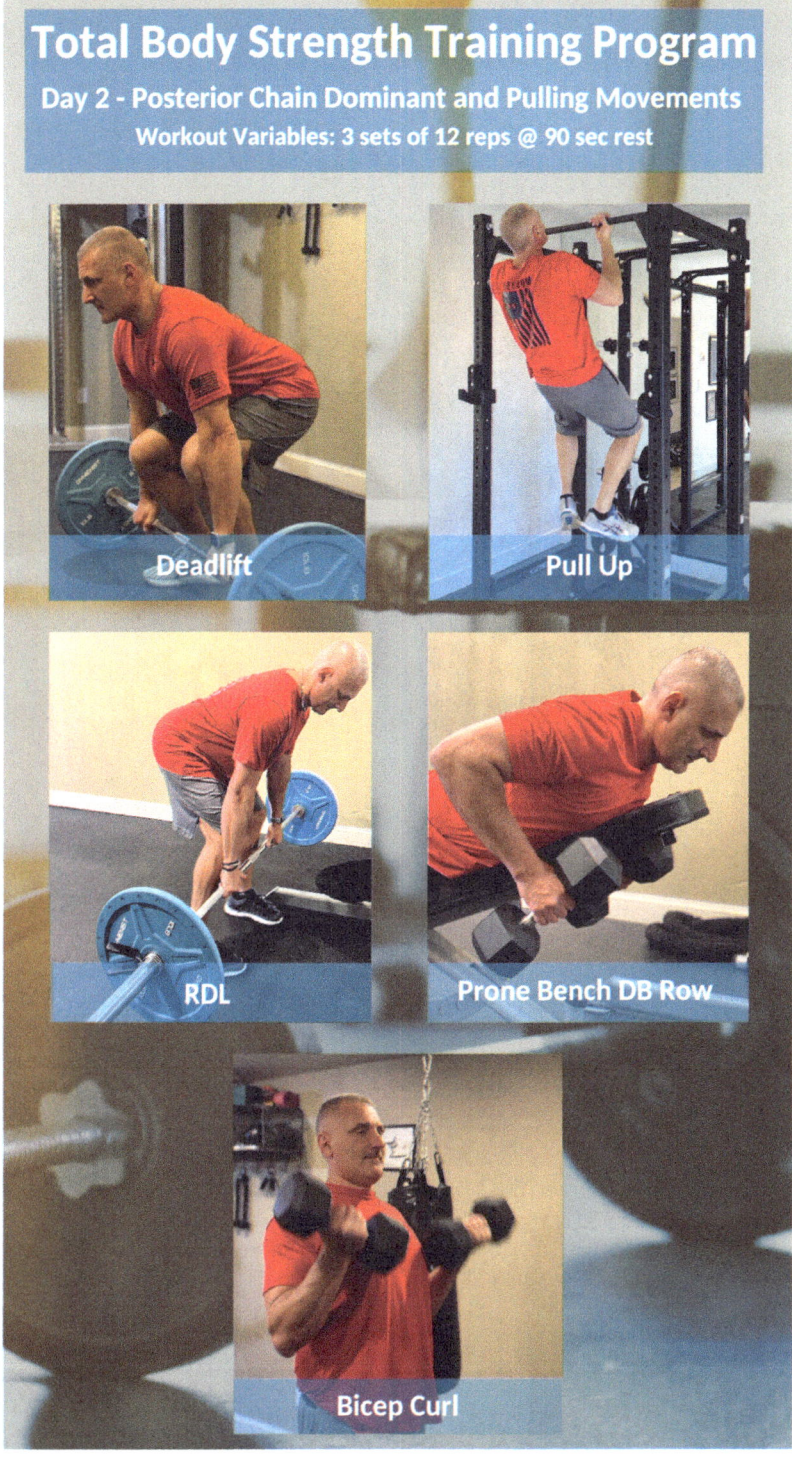

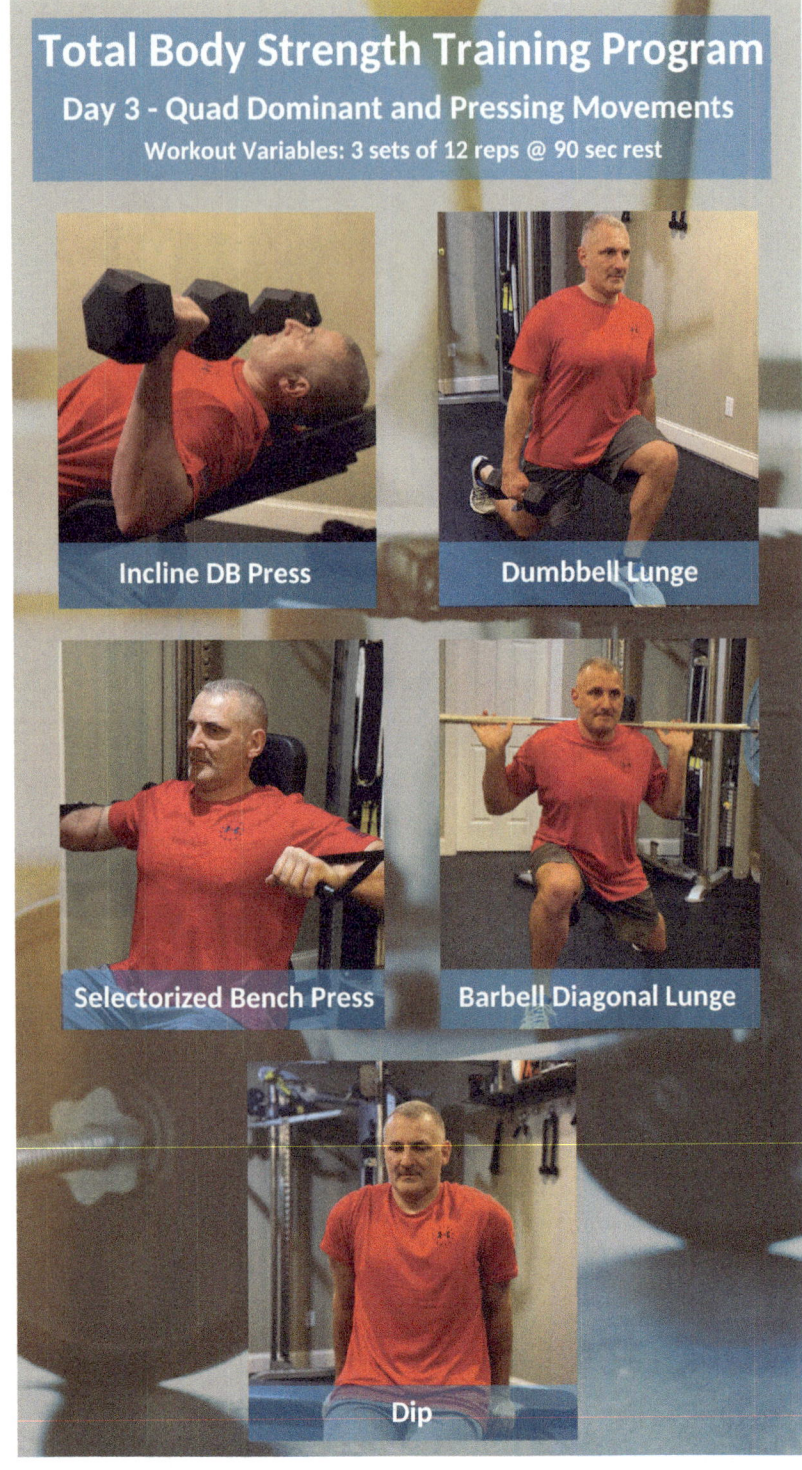

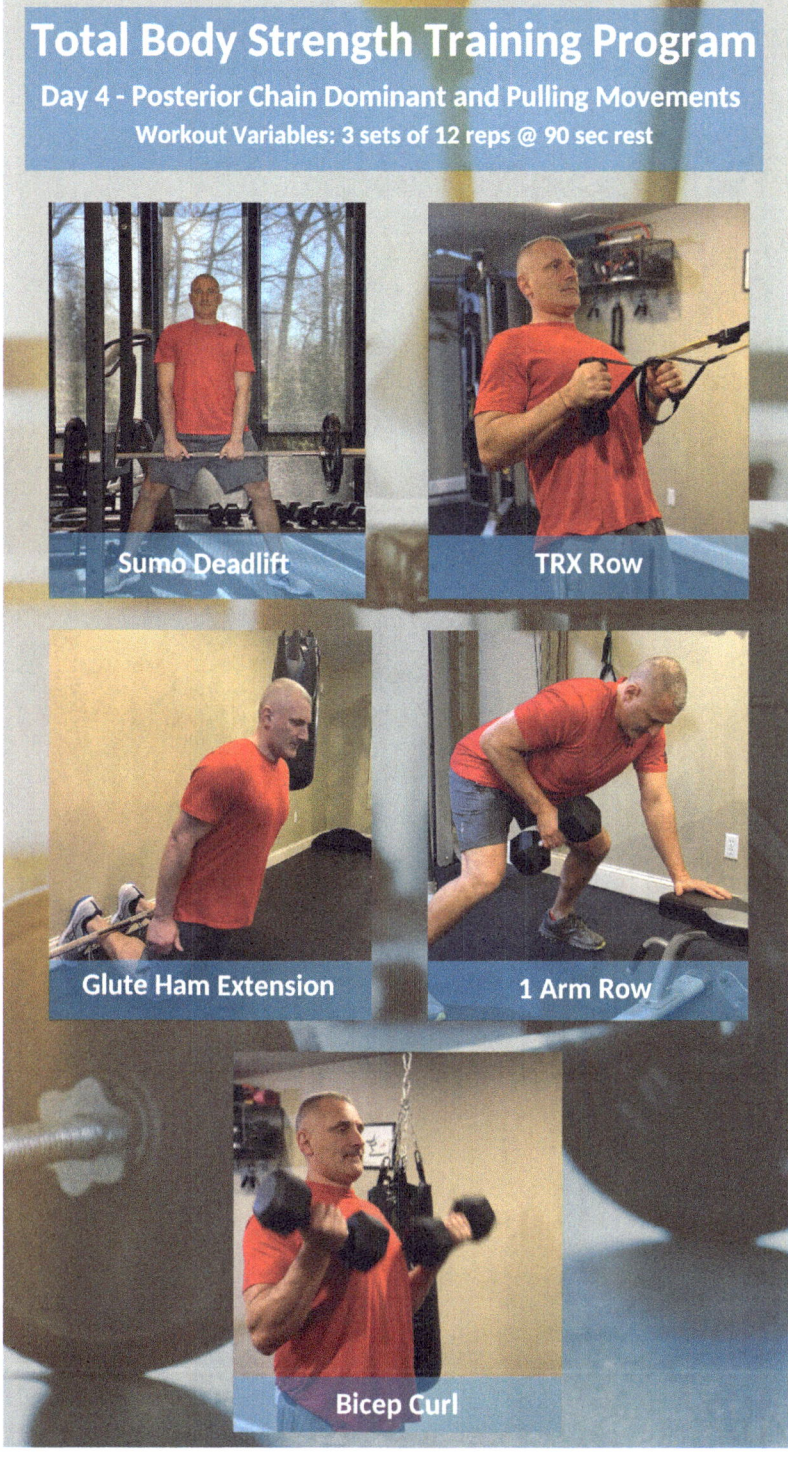

Bodybuilder Splits

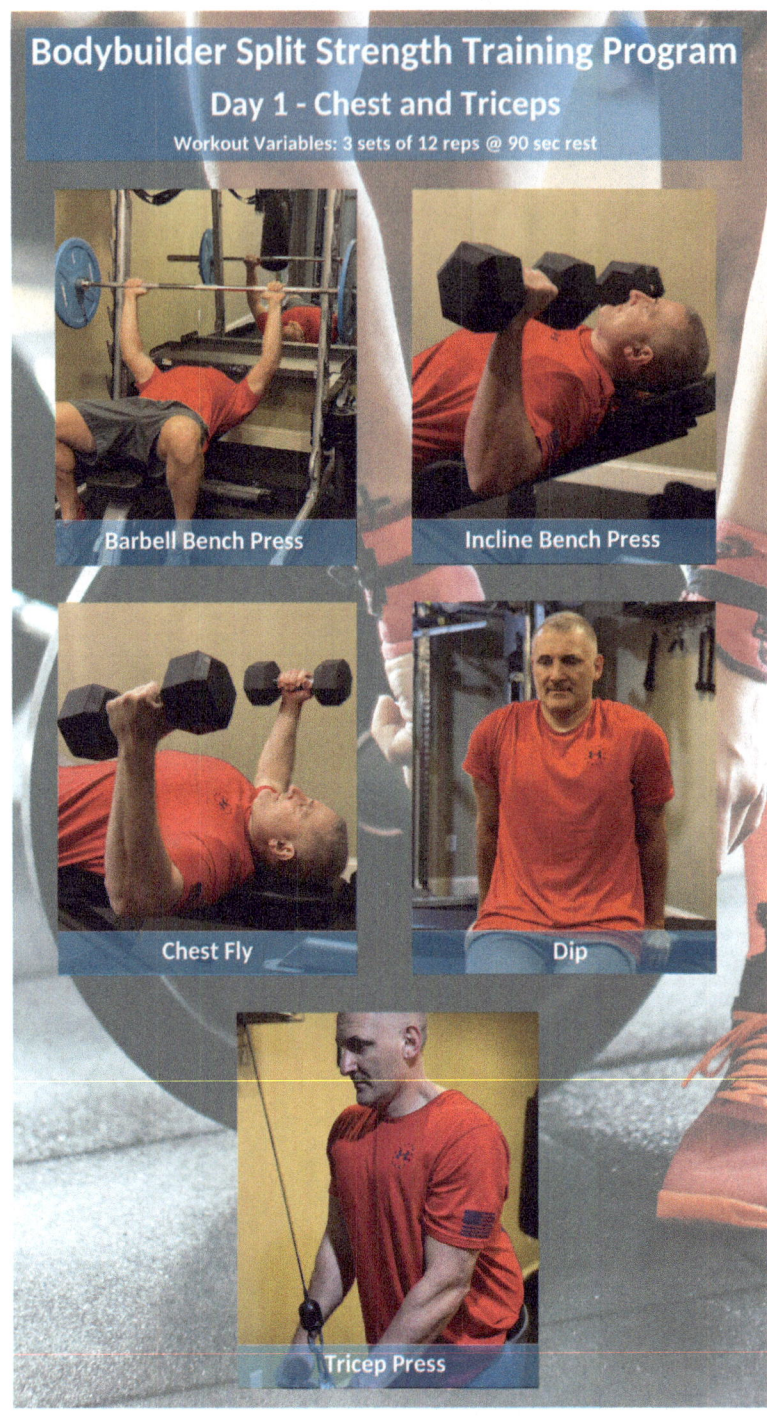

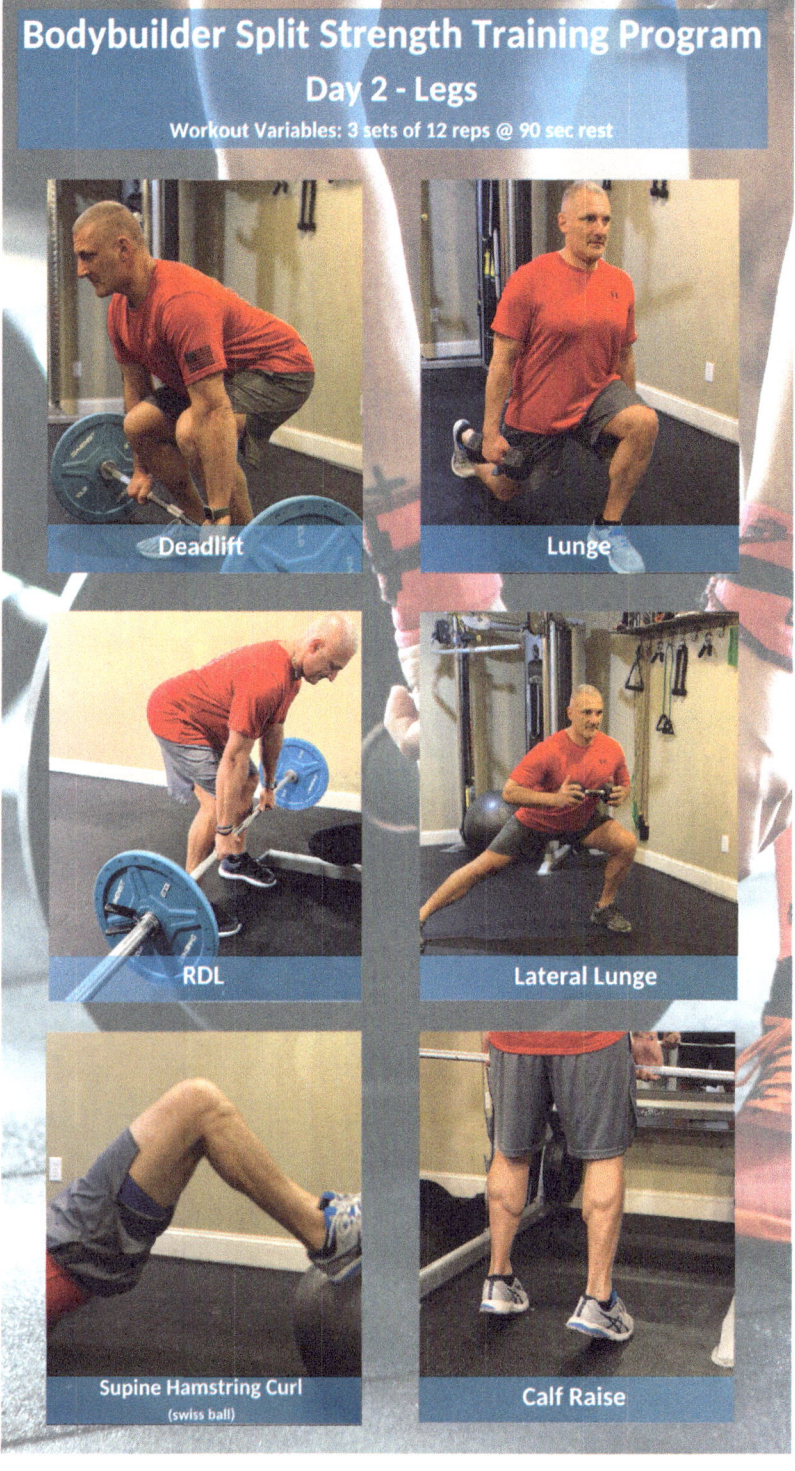

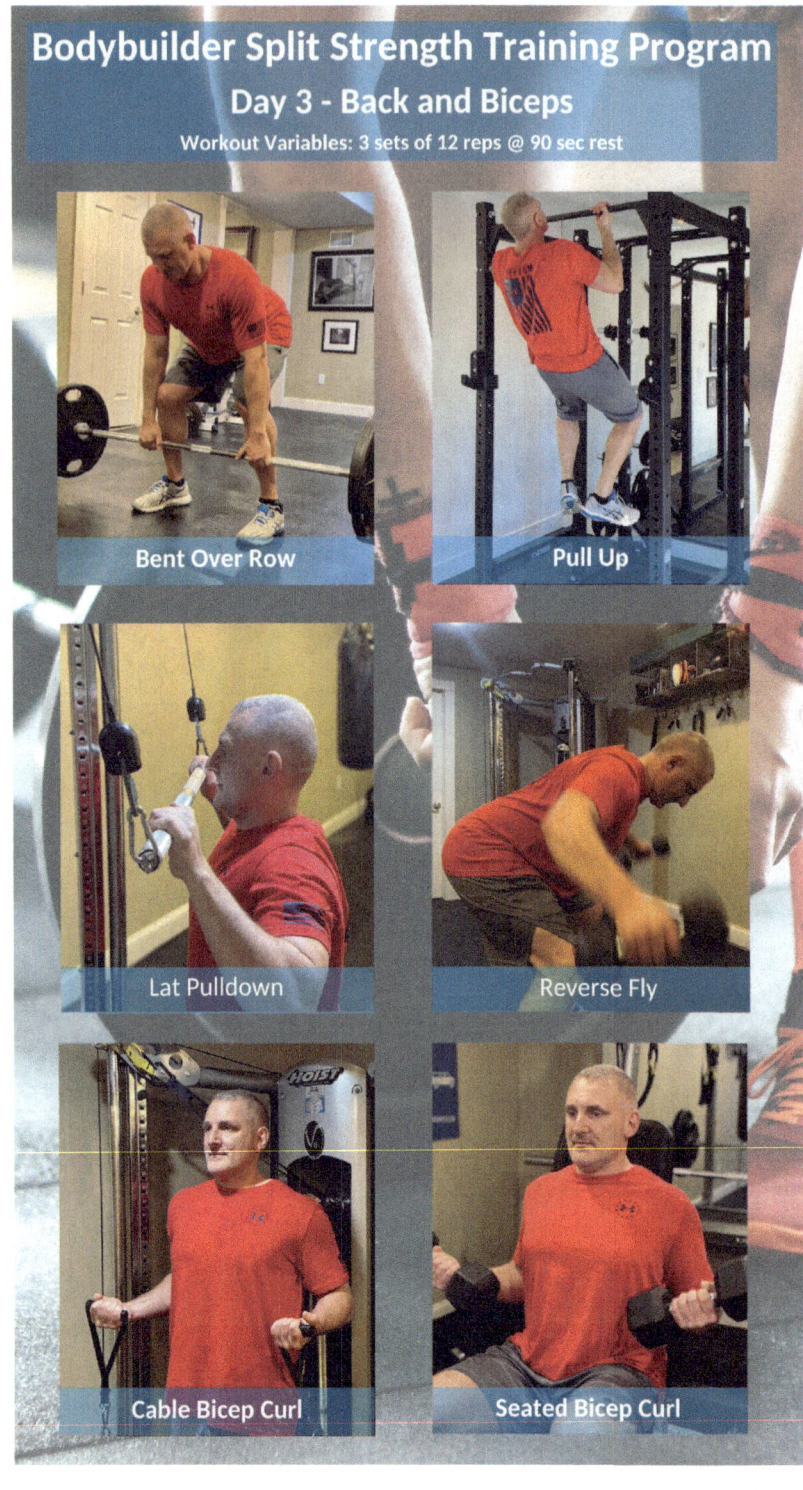

Supersets

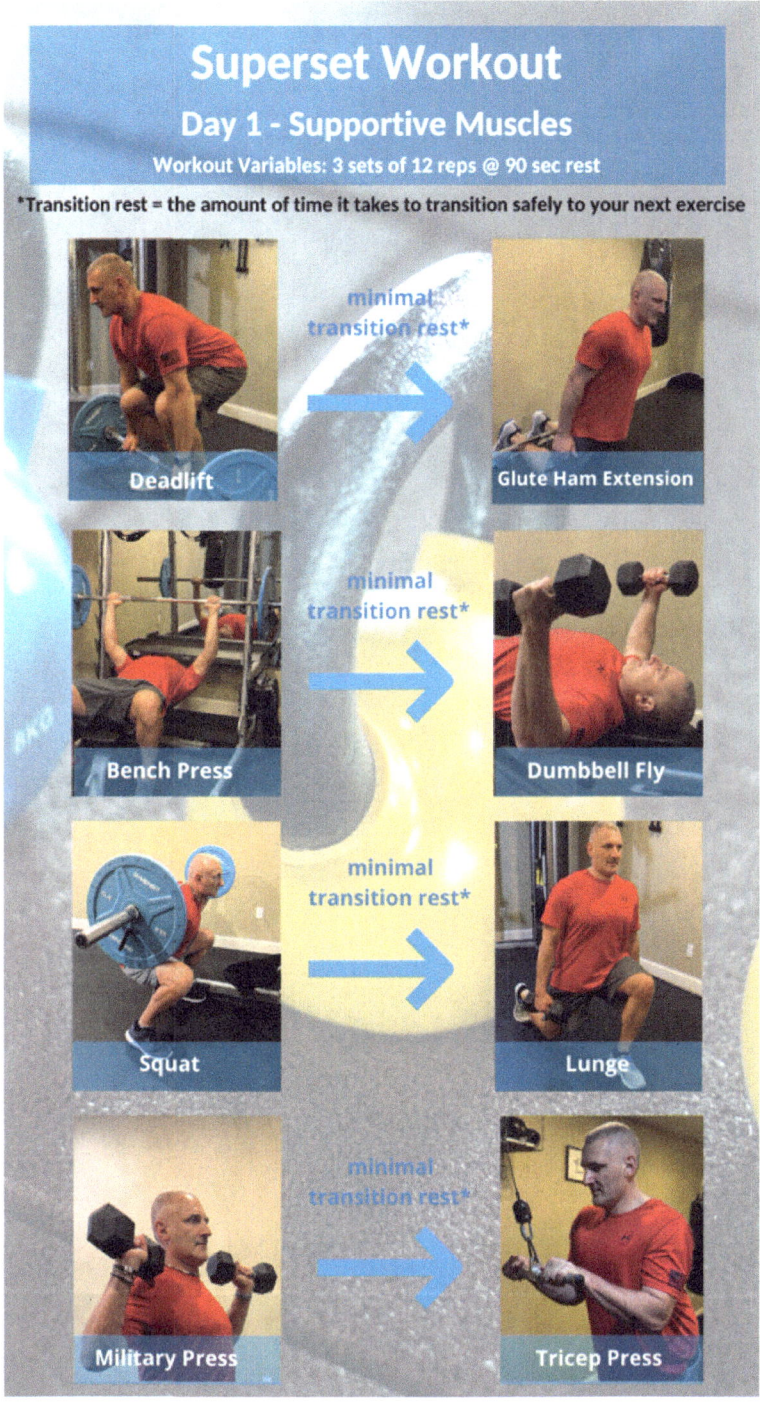

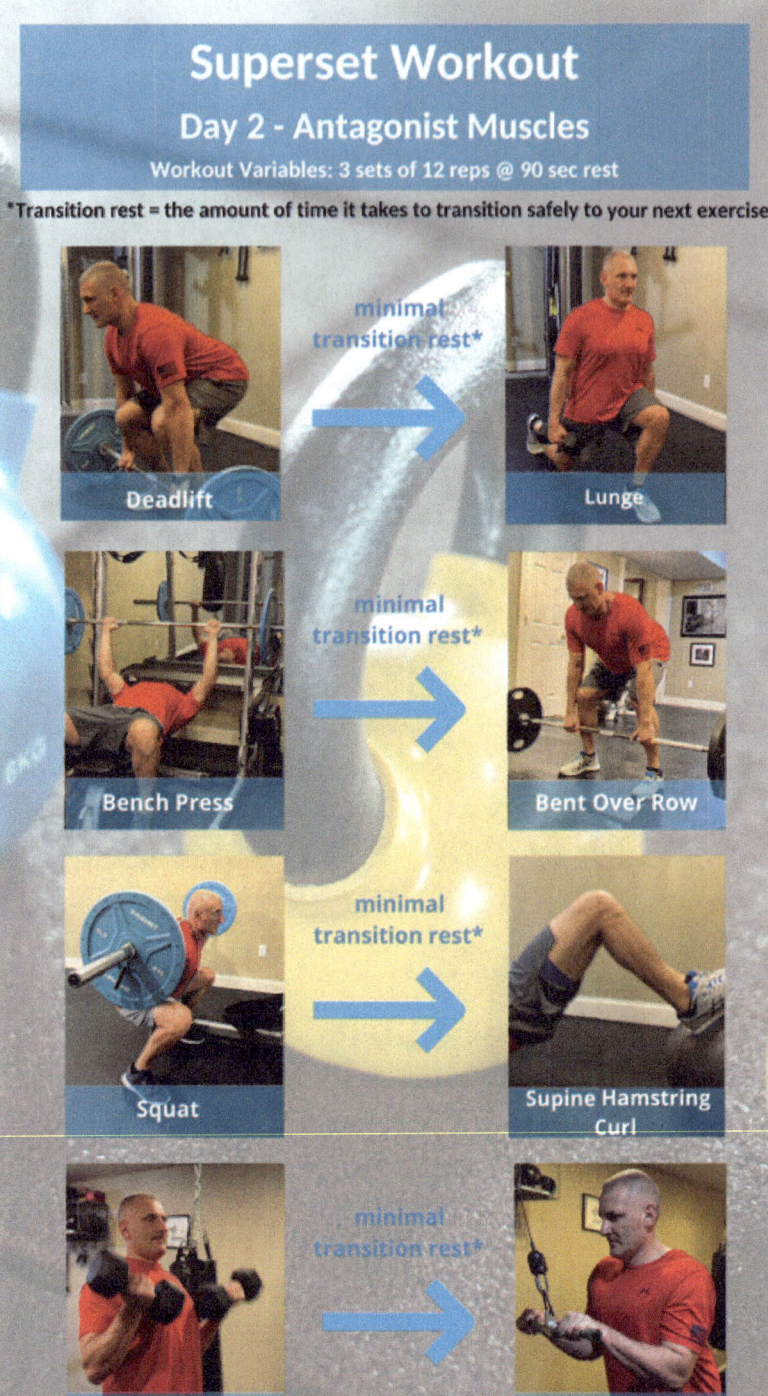

Power Training Upper and Lower Body

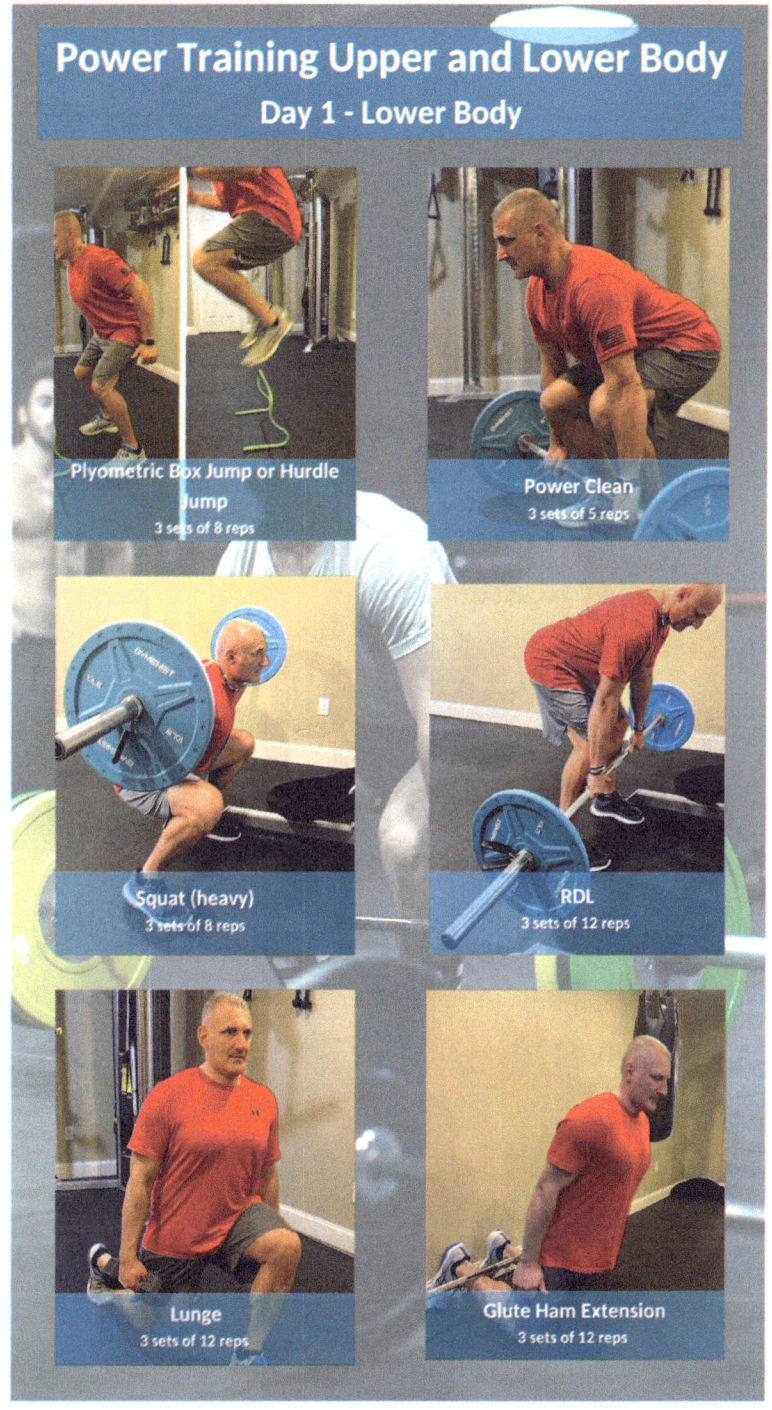

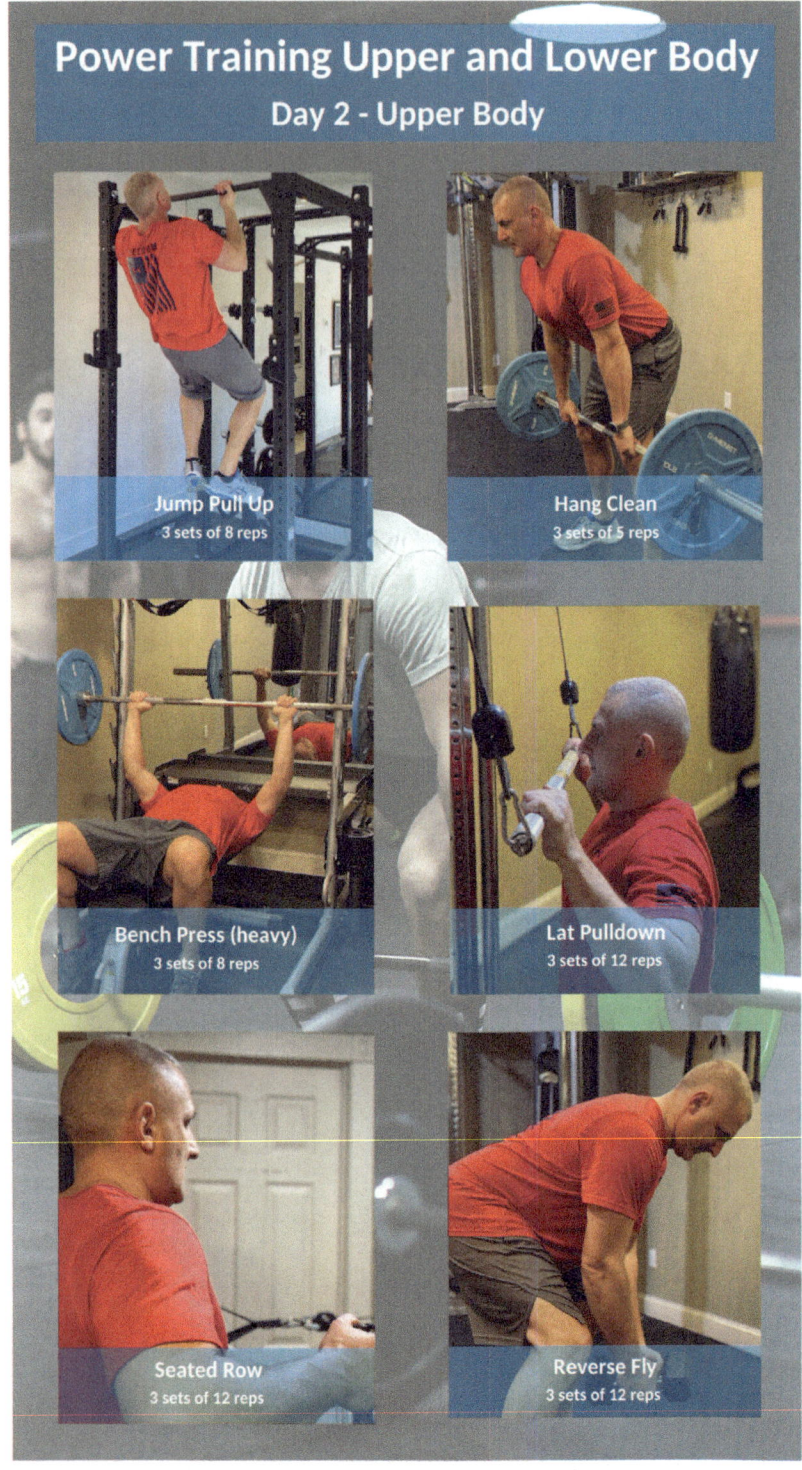

Home Gym (budget)

Home Gym Workout
Workout Variables: 3 sets of 12 reps @ 90 sec rest

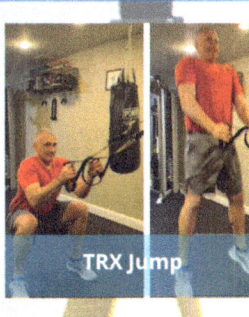
TRX Jump

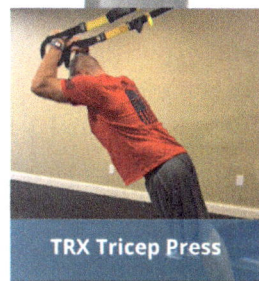
TRX Tricep Press

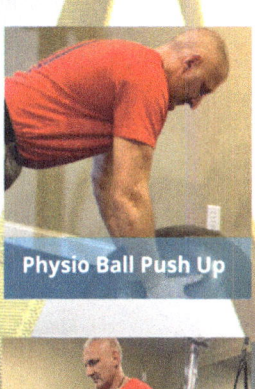
Physio Ball Push Up

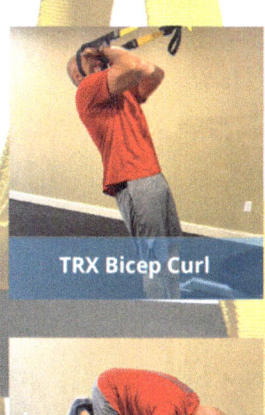
TRX Bicep Curl

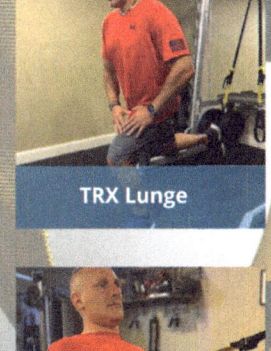
TRX Lunge

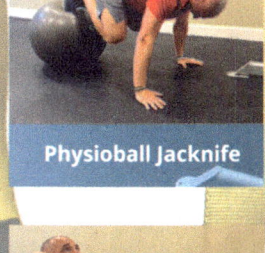
Physioball Jacknife

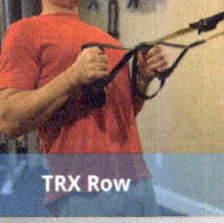
TRX Row

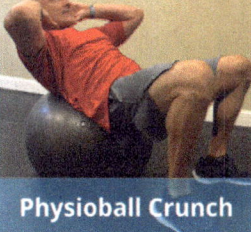
Physioball Crunch

Outdoor Workout

Outdoor Workout

 Workout variables: Cardio for 60 seconds followed by Strength for 90 seconds

- Warm-up = Walk or Jog (10 min)
- Band Walk to Right
- Band Walk to Left
- Jump Rope or Jumping Jacks
- Resistance Band Row
- Jump Rope or Jumping Jacks
- Walking Lunge
- Jump Rope or Jumping Jacks
- Standing Resistance Band Press
- Jump Rope or Jumping Jacks
- Resistance Band Squats
- Jump Rope or Jumping Jacks
- Resistance Band Bicep Curl
- Jump Rope or Jumping Jacks
- Bench Step Ups
- Jump Rope or Jumping Jacks
- Bench Dips
- Jump Rope or Jumping Jacks
- Cool down = Walk or Jog (10 min)
- Core at home

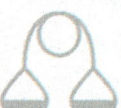
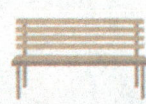

Beginners 101

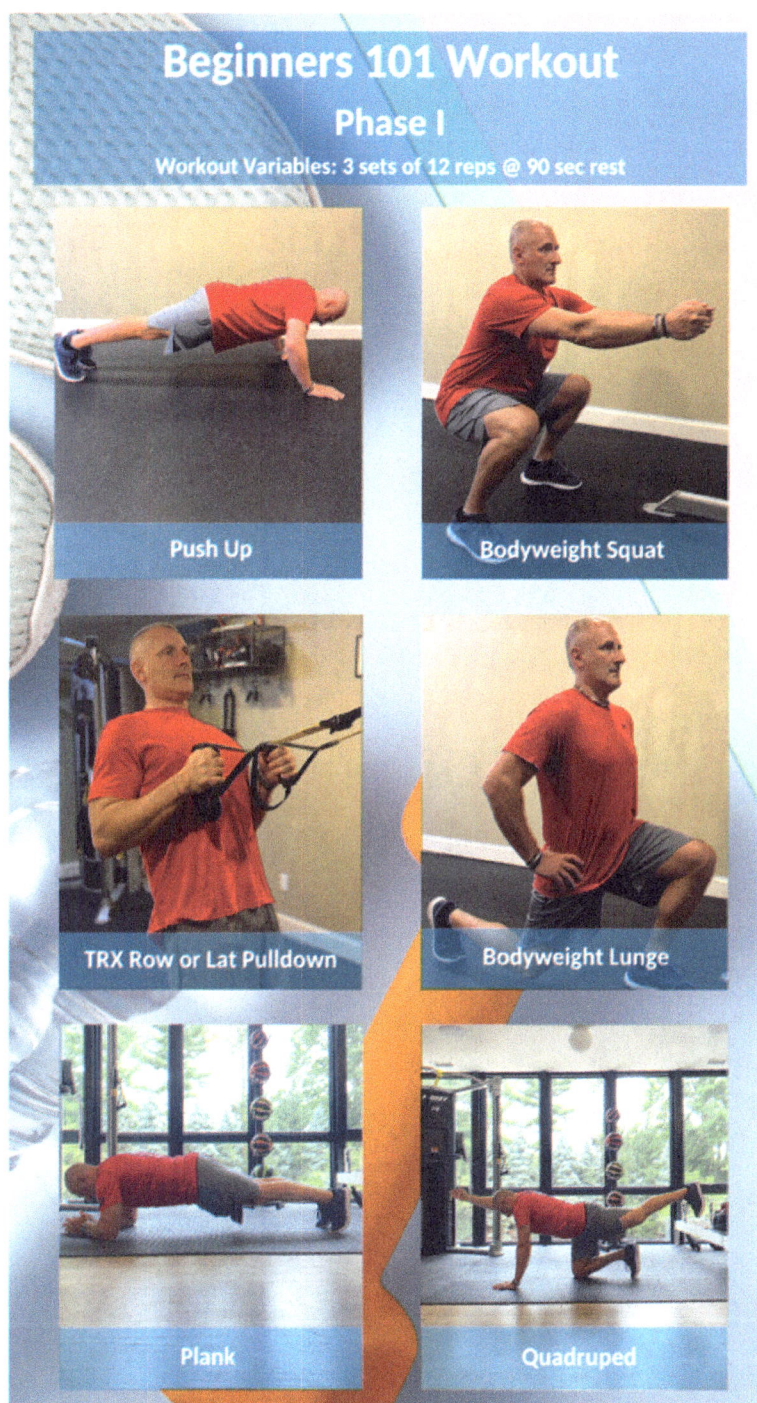

Beginners 101 Workout
Phase II
Workout Variables: 3 sets of 12 reps @ 90 sec rest

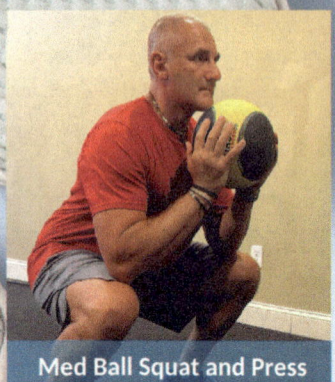
Med Ball Squat and Press

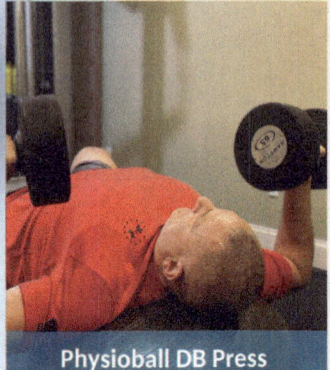
Physioball DB Press

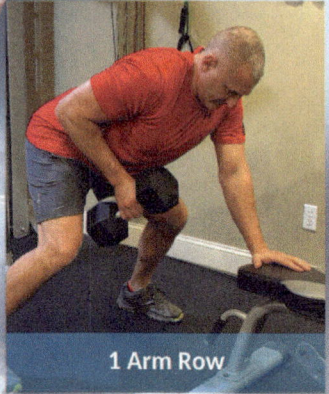
1 Arm Row

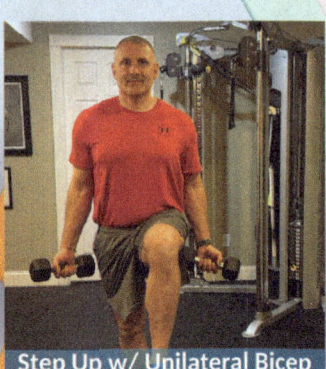
Step Up w/ Unilateral Bicep Curl into Press

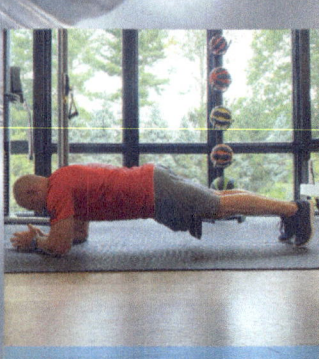
Plank Press

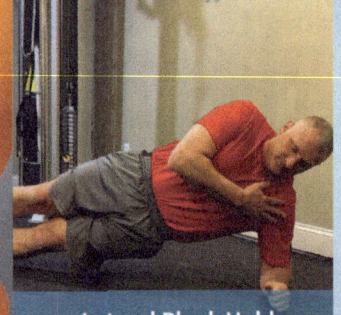
Lateral Plank Hold

Core

There are countless approaches and philosophies to addressing the core system. Below is a sample workout that can be used in combination with almost any workout. It utilizes a basic training principle I like to implement that addresses the key functions of the core system. You can substitute other exercises, but I'd recommend trying to match an appropriate exercise that reflects the category. For example, I reference a minesweeper as a functional exercise, you could easily substitute a Medicine Ball Wood Chop. Or for an isometric exercise, I use a front plank, you can easily substitute a lateral side plank. Also, similar to any strength program, there are countless ways to introduce sets, reps, weights, tempo, time under tension, external weights, etc. to provide a challenging stimulus.

A complete core program includes the following movement categories:

Functional - A movement that usually incorporates transmitting forces from the ground through the core and ending through the upper body. If you look at an athletic movement like throwing a baseball, the entire body is involved with the motion. Lying on your back and doing crunches won't prepare your body for that movement as well as a Functional Exercise.

Dynamic - Involves a contraction that moves the abdominal region in an intended range of motion. This is normally associated with isolated exercises aka "crunches" but can also be identified with more advanced exercises like hanging abdominal raises.

Isometric - A steady muscular contraction that occurs without either lengthening or shortening (contracting) of the muscles involved. As demonstrated by Stewart McGill and referenced earlier, essential underlying abdominal muscles are most effectively recruited with isometric movements. Planks are most identified with this category.

Posterior Chain - By definition this area references the glute, hamstring, and calf but we specifically want to target the glutes. Isolating the glute muscles can create an important sequential firing pattern that protects the back and builds and contributes to a strong core. However, if the glute doesn't fire properly more tension can be put on the back and or hamstring, which can create harmful stress on the core.

Injury Prevention - There are a whole array of movements that qualify as injury prevention including simply taking the program approach we are discussing now. However, the focus should really be on lighter movements that focus on balance, coordination, and proper muscle recruitment.

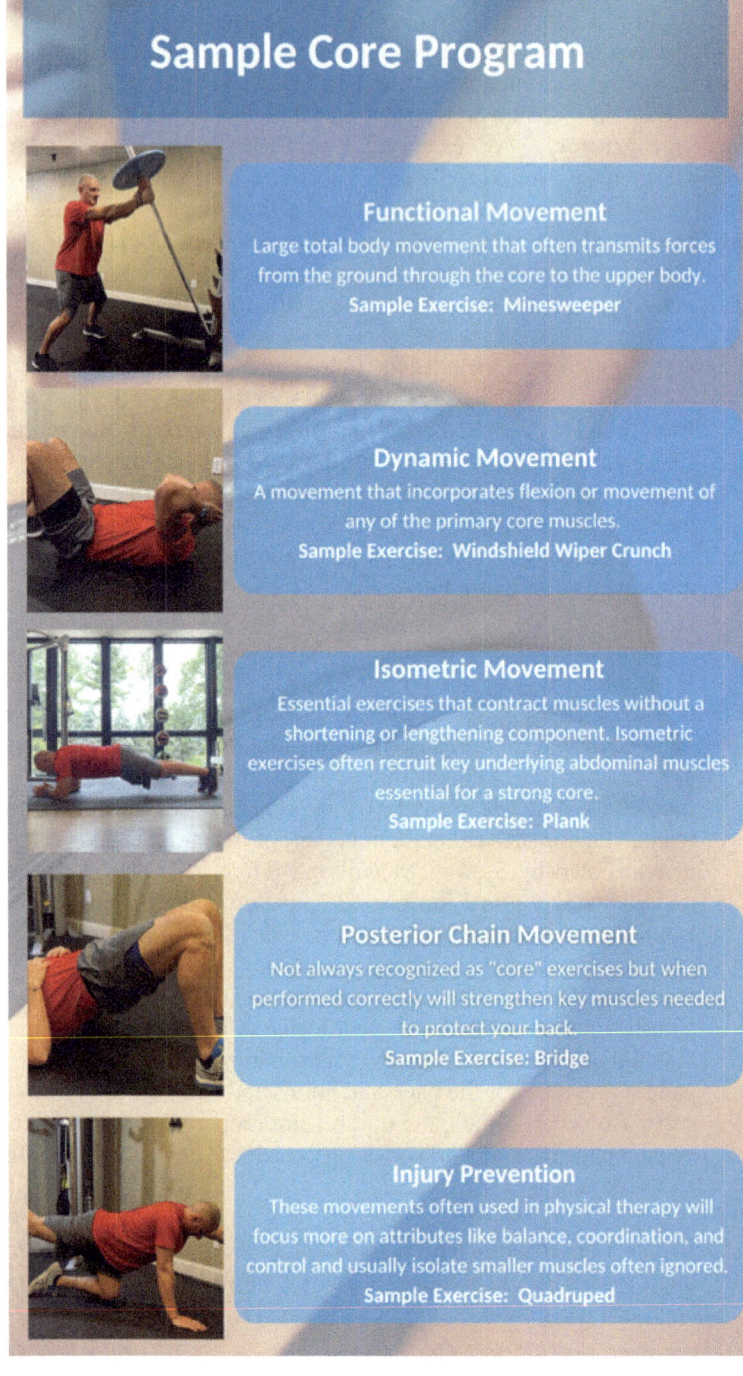

Sample Core Program

Functional Movement
Large total body movement that often transmits forces from the ground through the core to the upper body.
Sample Exercise: Minesweeper

Dynamic Movement
A movement that incorporates flexion or movement of any of the primary core muscles.
Sample Exercise: Windshield Wiper Crunch

Isometric Movement
Essential exercises that contract muscles without a shortening or lengthening component. Isometric exercises often recruit key underlying abdominal muscles essential for a strong core.
Sample Exercise: Plank

Posterior Chain Movement
Not always recognized as "core" exercises but when performed correctly will strengthen key muscles needed to protect your back.
Sample Exercise: Bridge

Injury Prevention
These movements often used in physical therapy will focus more on attributes like balance, coordination, and control and usually isolate smaller muscles often ignored.
Sample Exercise: Quadruped

I hope these workout examples offer some insight into the many options that are available for a strength training program. The ability to always change things up, and stimulate both your body and motivation, are key components to your success.

Post Workout Protocols

Cool Down- Try to add an additional 5-20 minutes of post cardio activity to your workout with the last few minutes at low intensity. You want to allow for your heart rate to slowly drop back to normal.

Static Stretch- Once you have completed your cool down cardiovascular activity, its a good idea and time to address tight or compromised areas with static stretching. Where static stretching can potentially negatively impact preparing for certain exercises, it is a great tool for assisting in your body's recovery.

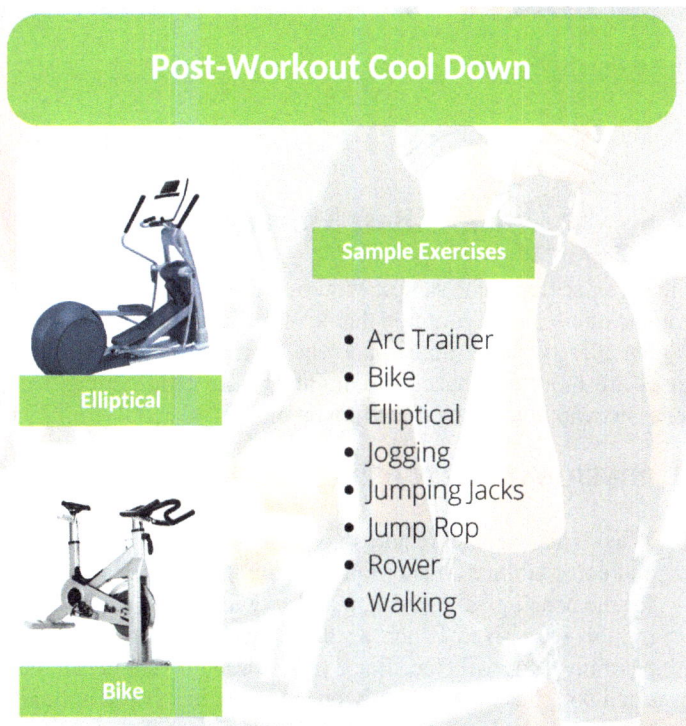

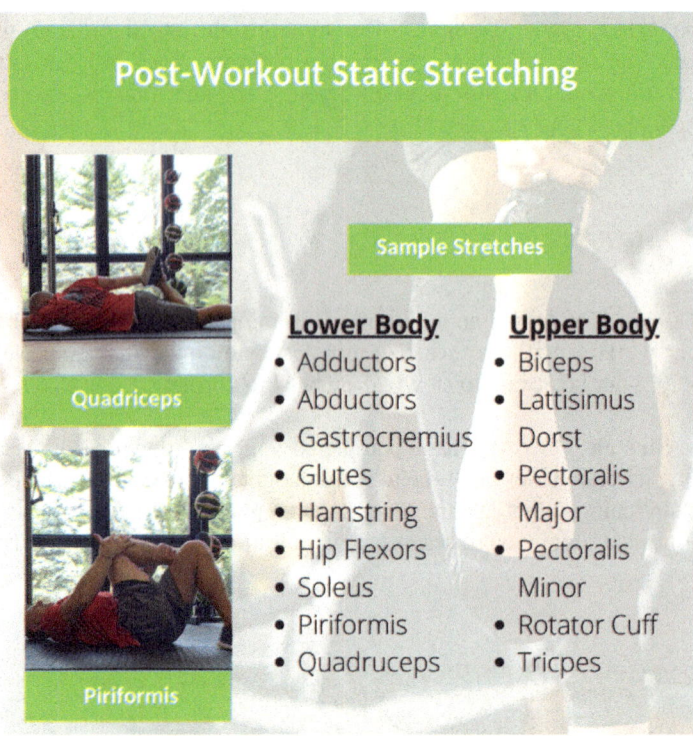

Top 5 Best Movements

Now that I've shared some sample workout designs, I want to share my top 5 favorite exercises. The common theme with all these exercises is that they are highly effective and functional when used properly. Most of these exercises are more advanced, so I highly recommend having a certified trainer assist you in learning these movements.

1. **PHYSIOBALL BENCH PRESS**

   Why- This exercise requires your entire body to engage in balance and core stability, in addition to firing the traditional muscles used for the bench press. Also, the ball provides a more natural range of motion vs a fixed bench as the ball contours to the body more naturally. You will sacrifice overall strength vs a bench barbell or dumbbell, but the total body engagement in what is normally seen as an upper body movement is worth it.

How- Align yourself on the ball so that your neck is perfectly contoured and widen your legs as much as needed to increase stabilization. Make sure all of your core muscles are engaged before beginning the pressing motion.

2. **STIFF-LEGGED DEADLIFT or ROMANIAN DEADLIFT (RDL)**

    Why- This movement is one of my favorite exercises, but probably one of the most dangerous movements to perform as the technique required is often not executed properly. However, when performed correctly it is a great posterior chain exercise and develops isometric lower back strength combined with hamstring and glute strength. I often tag this movement with a shrug and calf raise as these movements are usually done in an isolated fashion, which for me personally can be time consuming and not consistent with a total body training approach.

    How- The key to this movement is bending at your hips, "hinging", while not breaking neutral alignment of your spine or increasing range at your knee joint. The weight should be completely in the heel of the foot when descending. Focus on the bar coming toward the body and stop the descent when you are no longer pushing back through your hips.

3. **PULL UP**

    Why- While this is an extremely challenging movement, very few upper body exercises can match the intensity or results of this movement. Because of the difficulty, I recommend utilizing bands or machine assist to obtain more traditional repetitions. Meaning, most people can't do 3 sets of 12 repetitions of bodyweight pull ups, so offsetting your bodyweight is an important strategy when incorporating this movement into your workout.

    How- There are two grip options, over and underhand. When positioning your hands over or prone, align them past shoulder width (chin up). When positioning your hands underhand or supine, align your grip at shoulder width. Do your best to not rock or swing and try to pull through a full range of motion.

4. **SQUAT**

    Why- The squat is one of the most functional and demanding exercises out there. The fundamental movement pattern of raising your body from a seated to a standing position is as beneficial for an athlete as for a geriatric individual. It is one of the most functional patterns that we use in our lives, so creating an overload to strengthen all of the muscles used during this pattern is essential. A key component to this movement is learning how to develop and properly engage the core system to manage externally loading the spine. This is part learning how to maintain a proper spine (neutral alignment), and part learning how to engage and fire the core muscles that protect the spine.

How- Position your feet just past shoulder width and allow your feet to turn out slightly. Establish a comfortable spot across your shoulders to let the bar rest. Then descend, while maintaining a neutral spine, until you are able to go just below a parallel position. When descending, think of bending at your hips vs your knees and shifting the weight back into your heels vs leaning forward and shifting the weight to your knees.

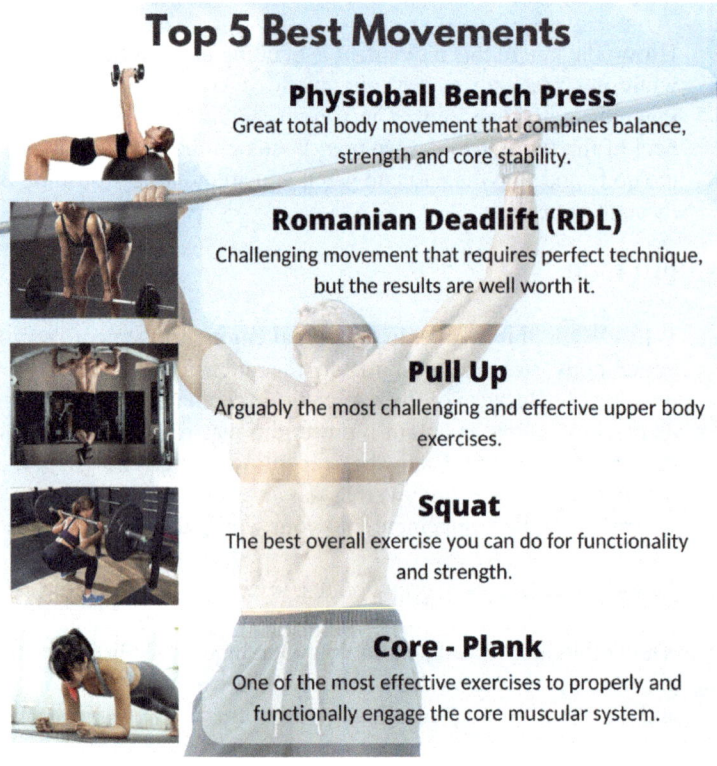

Top 5 Best Movements

Physioball Bench Press
Great total body movement that combines balance, strength and core stability.

Romanian Deadlift (RDL)
Challenging movement that requires perfect technique, but the results are well worth it.

Pull Up
Arguably the most challenging and effective upper body exercises.

Squat
The best overall exercise you can do for functionality and strength.

Core - Plank
One of the most effective exercises to properly and functionally engage the core muscular system.

5. *Core-* **PLANK**

Why- Teaching the core muscles to learn how to fire and properly brace to withstand opposing forces is the first step to developing a functional core. The core muscular system is complicated and has muscles that align parallel, perpendicular and diagonal to the spine. The muscles serve to both isometrically stabilize the spine as well as to functionally contract it. No movement better introduces your body safely to this movement than a plank.

How- Brace your entire core system, similar to what you would do if you were anticipating someone hitting you in the stomach. While this may seem extreme, it works to engage all of the necessary core muscles for this movement. Then align your body parallel to the ground, but as a tip, push your hips up slightly. It may feel like you are pushing your hips or butt out of alignment, but often we position with a slight sway. If possible, look in a mirror and assess if your back is straight or not.

Top 5 Exercises to Avoid

Working out is hard enough, but we also must accept that there is an inherent risk when externally loading your body. Knowing that there is risk of injury when performing good exercises, I'd like to help you stay clear of potential problems by at least avoiding the 5 exercises listed below. I feel these exercises can increase negative stresses to your body even when executed the way they were intended.

1. **SMITH MACHINE SQUAT**

    The smith bar runs on a linear tracking system, which restricts the ability of the body to move in a functional J like pattern while descending into a squat. Consequently, as the hip is unable to hinge and push the hips backward, the hips tuck under, forcing the spine into a non-functional position that can't properly distribute compressional loads. The irony here is that the smith bar is used as a safety piece of exercise but can actually increase back stress when used for squats.

2. **BEHIND THE BACK LAT PULLDOWN**

    Pulling a bar behind the back forces the shoulder to severely rotate, decreasing the functional space between the arm bone (humerus) and joint space (glenohumeral joint). Also, people often compensate by flexing their head forward to move it out of the way of the bar, which further misaligns the spine. To avoid this position, simply pull the bar to the front of the body or position your hands in a neutral (thumbs facing toward you) position by using a special bar or handles. A simple modification to your technique can change this from a shoulder wrecker to an effective exercise.

3. SEATED OVERHEAD TRICEP EXTENSION

This is a chain reaction movement. Seated with your hands positioned over your head often causes you to extend your spine due to hip flexor tightness. This position automatically puts stress at your lower back in addition to the weight load you are lifting. Then it often causes you to flex your head forward to help offset tightness and to create clearance when lifting the weight. This causes the potential to extend your lower spine and flex your cervical spine, neither of which match the goal of always having a neutral spine. Lastly, as the weight is lowered, excessive stress is placed on the shoulder joint, which can aggravate certain underlying shoulder conditions. There are too many ways to target the triceps, so avoid this unnecessary and potentially dangerous movement.

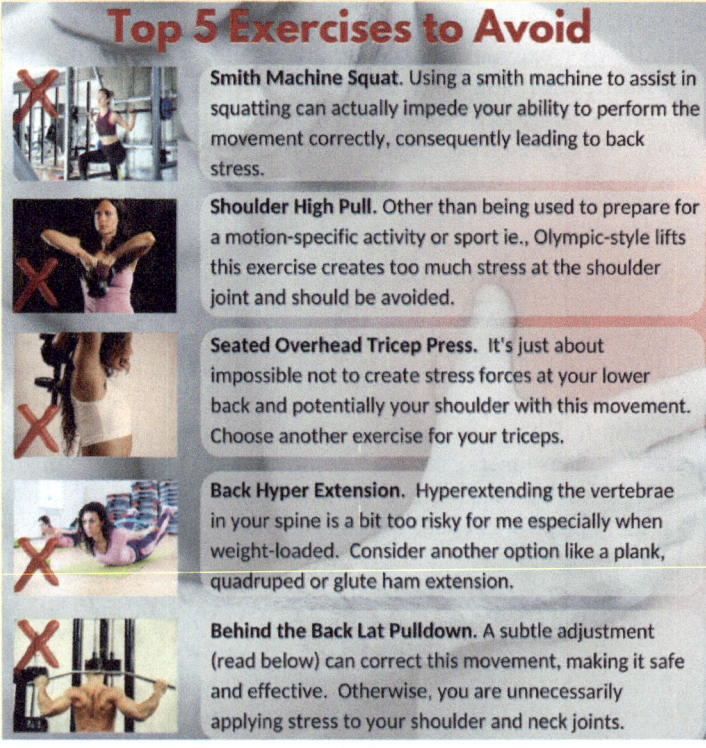

Top 5 Exercises to Avoid

Smith Machine Squat. Using a smith machine to assist in squatting can actually impede your ability to perform the movement correctly, consequently leading to back stress.

Shoulder High Pull. Other than being used to prepare for a motion-specific activity or sport ie., Olympic-style lifts this exercise creates too much stress at the shoulder joint and should be avoided.

Seated Overhead Tricep Press. It's just about impossible not to create stress forces at your lower back and potentially your shoulder with this movement. Choose another exercise for your triceps.

Back Hyper Extension. Hyperextending the vertebrae in your spine is a bit too risky for me especially when weight-loaded. Consider another option like a plank, quadruped or glute ham extension.

Behind the Back Lat Pulldown. A subtle adjustment (read below) can correct this movement, making it safe and effective. Otherwise, you are unnecessarily applying stress to your shoulder and neck joints.

4. BACK EXTENSION

While you can argue that the spine does need to have functional mobility, including extension, the idea of forcing extension can become dangerous. This is especially true when external loads, speed or additional movements are combined with the extension. The goal should be a functional fixed spine with the mobility taking place at the joints above and below it, namely the hip and shoulder. There are too many safe, functional and effective exercises to strengthen the back than to continue doing this movement, which can potentially hurt your back.

5. SHOULDER HIGH PULL

There is a specific range of motion known as the impingement zone, which is the area that injuries occur. This is roughly the exact range of motion that your shoulder will travel during this movement. Applying resistance during this exercise further increases stress to the shoulder joint. Now for those having fully healthy shoulders it's possible this movement may not cause you any discomfort, but why introduce a movement that is stressful to the joint if you don't have to.

At this point in the book, we've made a strong case that a smarter cardiovascular program, combined with an effective strength program, will boost your metabolism, allowing for your body to work harder for you instead of you working harder for your body! Specifically, we discussed that doing a HIIT cardio workout will burn more calories after your workout than traditional cardio training by eliciting the EPOC response. We learned that strength training will develop lean body mass, which consequently will increase your resting metabolic rate. So, combining these two strategies as the focus for your workouts will rev up your metabolism and help get you the results you are looking for. In our next chapter we will look at the third component of wellness, nutrition, and how it can also boost your metabolism if the right types of food are eaten.

Chapter 6:
Caloric Consumption and Nutrition

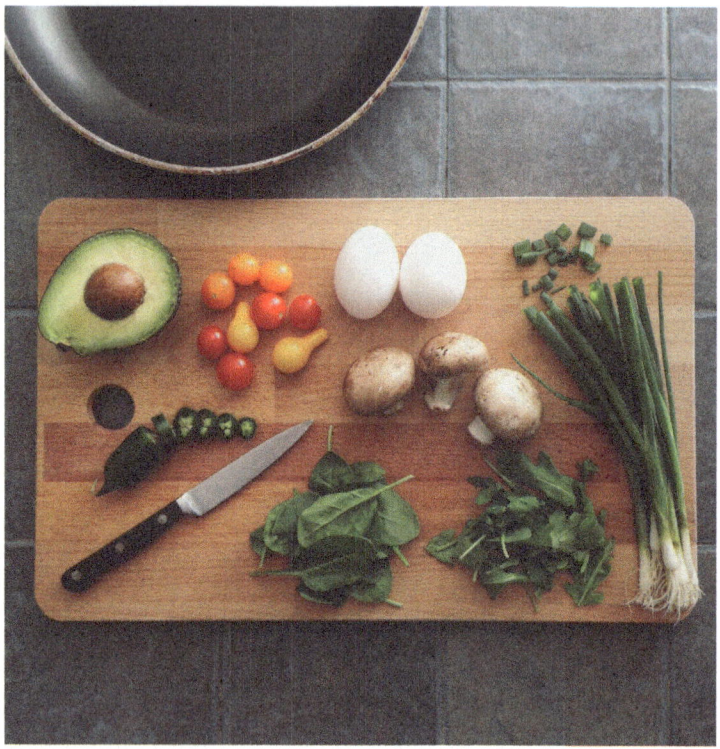

"Learn how to Eat Better, Not Less"
Dieting is out. Restriction is out. Fad diets are out. We know through sound scientific research that the "diet mentality" leads to rebound weight gain, disordered eating, injuries, chronic health conditions and most importantly lead to not feeling good!

What's in? Fueling our bodies with the nutrients it needs to feel our best, perform our best, look our best and be the healthiest version of ourselves that we can be for a long time to come.

The types of foods, the quantity and quality of the foods you choose, and the time at which you eat them can have a profound effect on weight loss. If the foods you eat provide you with better energy, satisfy your appetite, and allow you to enjoy what you are eating, then you have found the right nutritional plan for you. Ultimately, we want to stay away from the "Diet Mentality" and think along the lines of nutritional choices that provide the body with the fuel necessary to live actively.

Always remember that your body is unique. You have different needs based on your own metabolic rate, family history, health history, activity levels etc. You need to eat for your body. Don't fall into the trap of comparing yourself to others or eating the same way as others. Your food intake should always reflect your own personal needs and goals.

I spent the earlier part of my career in an all-girl independent school working with pre-teen and teenaged female athletes. It was at this time that I began to appreciate the devastating effects that body image and social pressure had on young girls. Consequently, I had to develop a more sensitive and creative approach to discussing nutrition as often their diets were flawed and contributing to a vicious cycle of empty calories and poor food choices. I had to discredit and discourage harmful strategies like "the calorie intake mindset" and shift their focus to assessing the benefits of the foods they were choosing. The caloric intake mindset of "a calorie is just a calorie" can justify Twizzlers and a diet soda as the same value as an apple. This is a problem that younger individuals often have trouble appreciating. As a way to better inform the girls at the school where I worked, I began to discuss their bodies in the context of athletic performance. Shifting the conversation away from aesthetics and focusing on functionality and performance allowed me to focus on attributes like getting stronger and faster with better food choices and the right physical conditioning. This positive, strong, and empowering view of their bodies and the nutrition needed to fuel them steered us away from the unhealthy images of bodies portrayed by the media.

This message is no different with adults. We need to look at food as a way to fuel our bodies to get stronger. In return, we will be healthier, reducing body fat and building lean body muscle, aka "looking better".

The focus should be on quality food choices vs quantity. People don't suffer from obesity by consuming too many fruits and vegetables. If you can improve the quality of your food choices, often the quantity won't be as much of an issue. In addition, if you are able to eat more quality meals over the course of a week, your body's ability to consume "cheat meals" is more tolerable. If you have 5 meals a day x 7 days a week, that's 35 quality meals. Adding 3 small desserts doesn't equate to a lot of damage when absorbed by the total amount of quality meals. However, if you are only eating 3 meals a day then those three cheat meals have a higher negative impact.

The perfect diet is a hoax! Recently I was asked by a client to explain how there can be so many different diets out there that actually seem to work? In my younger years, I would quickly dismiss many of these diets as fads preying on people's emotions and vulnerabilities rather than providing factual information that could lead to sustainable progress. I would challenge the long-term effectiveness of the diets and often point out a lack of scientific validity. Also, as I mentioned before, I'm opposed to the term "diet" which implies strict rules, limited food types, restricted amounts of calories, and a forced philosophy that can't possibly represent everyone. This approach contradicts my personal philosophy of making good nutritional choices to provide your body with the necessary nutrients to function.

However, I found myself going back to my client's question. There had to be something to learn from all of these diets and the positive impact they have demonstrated. I knew that most diets weren't supported by the scientific community, but they did demonstrate some degree of success from their subscribers. So, as I dug a bit deeper, I observed some similarities that I believe were their true reasons for success. In fact, there are similarities with many of the more successful diets and philosophies even though their ideologies differ.

Finding these successful strategies was a bit complicated because the themes of the diets can confuse you: avoiding carbs, avoiding fats, eating based on your blood type, eating the same way a certain geographic region does, consuming fruits and vegetables, no dairy, etc. So what are the common themes? I found that the most successful diet books/plans help you to become more conscious of the foods you are consuming. **Simply paying better attention to what you eat, how much, and how often can have a significant impact.** Being a conscious eater and being aware of what and why we eat something versus allowing poor habits, emotion, convenience, or sometimes pure boredom to dictate our eating habits will lead to bad food choices. Many of these diet plans provide logs to track foods and offer specific suggestions for food preparation, all of which went back to preparing nutrition in advance and being conscious of our choices.

So acknowledging some of the positive lessons from the "diet crazed" market, let's focus on the science and begin to provide the necessary information that will allow you to make good food choices and be more conscious of what you eat.

First, the simple science of weight gain is that 3,500 calories = one pound. If you maintain an adequate balance of activity with intake you will maintain your weight. If your balance falls behind and your intake exceeds your activity level, you gain weight or vice versa.

So how do you know how many calories you should be consuming? If you are relying on what feels right or your caloric intake from younger years, then you may be in trouble. As mentioned earlier, many people will suffer a natural (though reversible) decline in necessary caloric requirements as their metabolism decreases with age. The most effective way to estimate your caloric intake is to have an accurate body fat analysis to determine your lean body mass. **Your lean body mass is what determines how many calories you need at rest to sustain itself.** Activity levels and types of food consumed have an impact on your overall caloric expenditure beyond your base levels. Once you know how many calories your body needs to sustain itself, you need to have an appreciation for how many calories you are consuming.

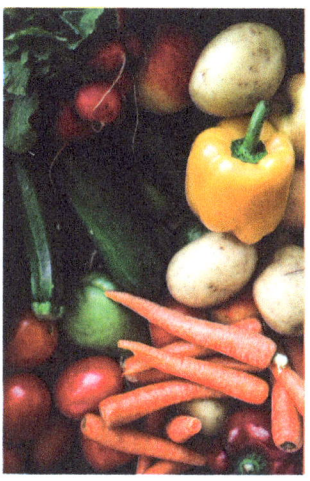

Carbohydrates and protein provide 4 calories per gram while fat has 9 calories per gram. However, this doesn't account for the thermic effect (discussed below) of food and the negative effect of artificial sweeteners. The point is that simply counting calories does not tell the whole story.

People aren't always aware that just by making better food choices you can actually burn more calories. This is a result of the energy required by your body to break down the food and digest it. **This phenomenon is called the thermic effect of food.** The nutritional intake, breakdown, and digestive process burn roughly 10% of the total calories consumed based on the types of food you eat. This is an unbelievable concept for a lot of people to learn and is an extremely effective strategy in a wellness plan.

To further enhance this effect, try to consume small frequent meals (5-7) a day. This will allow this effect to take place multiple times during the day and improve your total calories burned. If you only consume a few large meals the results won't be as effective as only so many calories can be stored efficiently. Many of the leading diets utilize some interpretation of this concept and its effect.

So which foods best utilize the thermic effect of food and why? As a general rule, foods that aren't processed and are low in sugar yield a higher thermic effect. Consequently, you will burn more calories from eating these foods. Try to visualize a piece of white bread and a handful of almonds, if you put them both into a fishbowl, which do you think would dissolve or break up first? It seems pretty straight forward that the bread would break down the quickest, right? This example is only further exaggerated in the complex digestive system which ultimately has to take solid foods and break them down to small enough particles to be absorbed into our bodies for nutrients or removed as waste.

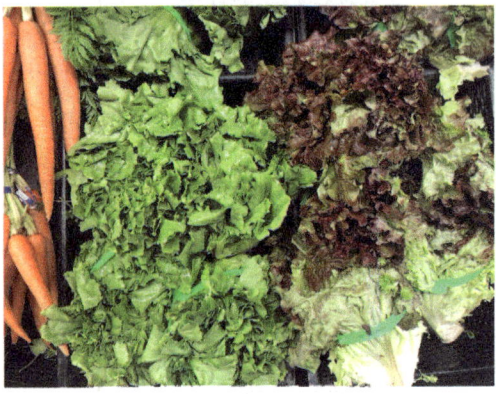

Protein and foods high in fiber (fruits and vegetables) are both very effective at increasing the thermic effect or slowing the digestion of foods. Lean protein foods can burn an additional 20-30% of the initial calories consumed. Therefore, **eating small meals throughout the day and focusing on fruits, vegetables, and lean proteins is an effective strategy to enact the thermic effect.**

In addition to understanding the thermic effect of food, another important concept to understand is blood sugar regulation. Choosing whole foods and balancing meals with complex carbohydrates, lean protein and good fat will help you maintain a steady blood sugar response. The importance of this is to avoid insulin spikes and hence subsequent fat storage. Regulating your blood sugar, along with increasing the thermic effect of food will speed up your metabolism, help build lean muscle mass, avoid fat storage and increase the amount of energy you feel!

If you recall during **Chapter 2: Why People are Failing at Fitness**, we identified sugar as enemy #1 and not fat. Poor nutrition often lies in excessive consumption of sugar, which is the true killer. Sugar delivers empty calories, rarely leaves you satiated, and creates havoc on your hormonal response to digestion. It leads to weight gain, health issues, and poor energy levels. Sometimes misfortune can teach us some very valuable lessons, for example individuals that develop diabetes are often forced to eliminate processed carbs and sugars from their diets. In many instances, these individuals will transform their bodies simply as a result of reducing or eliminating simple carbohydrates and replacing them with healthier food choices.

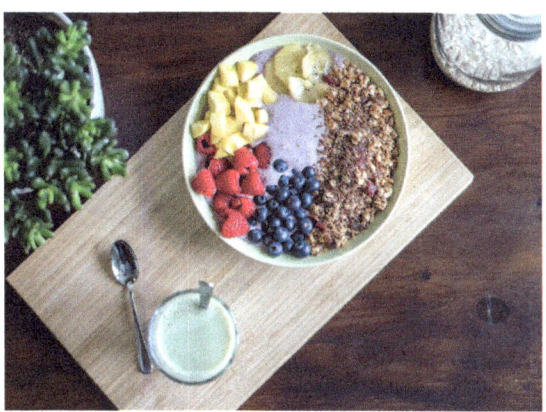

Fats are good! It's still crazy to me how misunderstood the consumption of fat has been for so many years in this country. We used to consider fat as the culprit to weight gain and heart disease. We now know that the type of fat we consume is crucial to our overall health. Knowing what types to eat regularly and which ones to limit is key.

Unsaturated fats assist in many functions in your body. They are crucial for brain function, joint health, organ protection, inflammation control, cholesterol management, optimize hormone balance, and assist in building strong muscles and bones. Fats help us feel full and help with the absorption of fat-soluble vitamins. They are often more satiating and consequently can help control appetite. "Good Fats" aka unsaturated fats increase the production of HDL (aka good cholesterol) and serve to help clear the arteries of build-up that creates blockages. "Bad Fats" aka Saturated fats, increase LDL, (aka bad cholesterol) which contributes to plaque buildup and obstruction along the walls of the arteries. Bad cholesterol levels block the opening of the arteries, restricting nutrients and oxygen to our vital organs. Eventually, this can lead to blockage in our arteries, which leads to heart disease. If the blockages are created in arteries that serve the brain it results in stroke.

There are 4 types of fat: saturated, polyunsaturated, monounsaturated, and hydrogenated (trans fats).

Saturated fats are recognized as bad fat and can contribute to artery obstruction. They are solid at room temperature and are found in the greatest quantities in animal products such as full fat dairy, fatty meats, and processed foods such as baked goods, crackers, chips etc. Saturated fats in moderation are fine (less than 10% of fat consumption). They provide benefits for brain function, protein for muscle, assist in the bone-building process, and provide higher levels of satiation.

Examples:
- beef
- lamb
- pork
- dark meat poultry
- whole milk
- full fat cheese
- butter
- full fat ice cream
- coconut and coconut oil
- lard
- shortening
- palm oil and palm kernel oil

Polyunsaturated fats are good fat. They are liquid at room temperature and are found in vegetable oils such as avocado, sunflower, and corn. These fats have the opposite effect of saturated fats as they can lower cholesterol. In addition to helping with cholesterol, they provide essential fatty acids, specifically the well-publicized Omega-3 fatty acid. Among other things, Omega 3 fatty acids reduce the blood's tendency to clot thus helping to prevent heart disease and stroke. *Think back to the hose and picture a solution actually stopping the plaque buildup along the* arterial walls.

Examples:
- walnuts
- sunflower seeds
- flax seeds or flax oil
- fish: salmon, mackerel, herring, albacore tuna, trout
- corn oil
- soybean oil
- safflower oil

Monounsaturated fats are another good fat. They are usually liquid at room temperature but may harden when cooled. These good fats share many of the positive properties of polyunsaturated fats. These fats are the basis for the Mediterranean Diet and suggest that a healthy consumption of these fats reduces many of the heart and health issues found in the U.S.

Examples:
- olives
- olive oil
- avocados
- almonds
- cashews
- peanuts

Hydrogenated or Trans Fats are man-made fats and are the worst form of fat out there. Technically they are unsaturated fats that have been chemically altered by adding hydrogen to them. They were created to help preserve foods longer and to be more cost-effective with cooking and frying foods. These fats have been shown to have more of a negative impact on cholesterol than saturated fats by lowering good cholesterol and raising the bad. Note: On the ingredients label of products, you will find these fats listed as "hydrogenated oil" or "partially hydrogenated oil".

Examples:
- cakes
- cookies
- some granola bars and protein bars
- pie crusts
- potato, corn, and tortilla chips
- deep-fried food: french fries, doughnuts, and fried chicken
- canned biscuits and cinnamon rolls, frozen pizza crusts
- non-dairy coffee creamer
- margarine

Our attempts to avoid fat have led to multiple pitfalls including increased consumption of sugar-free soda and artificial sweeteners, which ironically leads to increased weight gain and increased risk for other health issues. I realize this is counter-intuitive, but artificial sweeteners are hundreds to thousands of times sweeter than regular sugar, activating our genetically programmed preference for sweet taste more than any other substance. They trick our metabolism into thinking sugar is on its way. This causes our body to pump out insulin, the fat-storage hormone, which lays down more belly fat. It also confuses and slows down our metabolism, so you burn fewer calories every day. It makes you hungrier and you crave even more sugar and starchy carbs like bread and pasta.

Ultimately, proper nutrition and moderation are key, so if you need to use a sweetener, you are better off using a little sugar. **Balanced nutrition with sources found in their natural state will make you feel and look better, have better energy, and a more controlled appetite.** This process doesn't happen overnight but is experienced gradually, just like in fitness when you change your habits.

Nutritional Guidelines:

- **Eat every 2-3 hours with a goal of 5-8 smaller meals per day.** Remember the thermic effect of food and how it can increase your metabolism by up to 20% based on the quality of foods you consume.

- **Eat complete meals trying to focus on lean proteins and having either a fruit or vegetable with each meal.**

- **Eat complex carbohydrates like whole grain rice, fruits, and vegetables.** Remember simple sugars/ carbohydrates are what lead to weight gain.

- **Ensure that 25-35% of your energy intake comes from fat, primarily from monounsaturated (e.g., olive oil), and polyunsaturated (e.g. flax oil, salmon oil).** Remember fats will not make you fat. Healthy fats provide a multitude of health benefits.

- **Be conscious of the dangers of sugar and fat-free options in your diet and choose in moderation.** As discussed before, fat-free normally means more sugar or chemical sugar substitutes. Neither is good for the body.

- **Eliminate zero-calorie sodas and fat-free ice cream** and limit the use of sports drinks like Gatorade when using it as a sports supplement. Water and green tea are better options. (*Tip: Flavoring water with lemon or cucumber can be a great way to make water more enticing if you get bored of plain water.*)

- **Eat mostly whole foods.** The best diet tip I have ever heard is to "eat it if it came from the ground or had eyes". By saying "eyes", I'm really encouraging fish and lean animal options. In other words, whole fruits and vegetables coupled with lean protein. Avoid processed foods especially sugars and trans fats.

- **Try to consume at least one of these options with every meal:**
    - **Salmon** is good for your heart, skin, and brain. A great source of protein and is full of omega-3 fats. (*Tip: Choose wild salmon or organically farmed salmon to ensure the best quality.*)
    - **Green leafy vegetables** are great sources of iron, folate, and antioxidants. Kale has become the superstar of this group. It is loaded with cancer-fighting antioxidants and is high in fiber and Vitamin K and thus is on most experts' "superfood list". (*Tip: Adding kale or spinach to smoothies*

or dicing them up and adding them to a stir fry or a grain dish is an easy and effective way to boost nutrient intake in your day!)

- **Eggs** are high in protein and an important nutrient for brain health. Research has lightened on the negative effects of the yolk on cholesterol, but moderation and consumption of the egg white are a great option. (*Tip: Hard boil eggs each week for a simple and healthy nutrient rich grab and go option.*)
- **Fruits and Vegetables**. A variety of fruits and vegetables will never steer you wrong. Also, while fresh is preferable, frozen is better than nothing. Fun Fact: **Actually in many cases frozen veggies have a higher nutritional profile because they are flash frozen when they are harvested vs sitting on a truck for a few days before making it to the grocery store produce section. Buying fresh produce at a farmers' market is best, but don't fear frozen fruits and veggies as a convenient back up!
- **Avocados** offer an abundance of fiber and heart-healthy monounsaturated fats, plus antioxidants. (*Tip: Add sliced avocado to sandwiches, diced avocado to salads, or smashed avocado to dip veggies in as an appetizer!*)
- **Nuts**
    - Walnuts are healthy fats that are high in fiber, protein, and essential vitamins and minerals.
    - Almonds are high in protein, fiber, and antioxidants.
- **Lentils, Chickpeas, and Beans** are high in fiber and protein. (*Tip: Make hummus with chickpeas, prep Lentil soup early in the week for an easy and protein filled lunch option, add beans to stews or a grain-based side dish.*)
- **Greek yogurt** is a high protein source and a good quality source of complex carbs. (*Tip: Replace Greek yogurt for sour cream on taco Tuesday! Make a yogurt parfait with granola, fruit and nuts for a balanced energy producing breakfast or add it to a smoothie to boost protein content.*)
- **Sweet potatoes, and Potatoes** are a great source of energy and vitamins. Fun Fact: **Red potatoes have a more favorable blood sugar response than other potatoes. Roasting them with olive oil, sea salt and herbs brings out their wonderful flavor and makes a great addition to any balanced meal. (*Tip: Adding roasted and diced sweet potatoes to a salad can enhance the carbohydrate content of the salad (most salads are void of carbs). They create a great flavor and are more satiating than a side of bread.*)

- **Quinoa and Kamut** are grains that are high in protein and fiber. (*Tip: Try new grains! Barley, Buckwheat, Bulgar Wheat, Millet, Oatmeal are all wonderful sources of complex carbs and you can incorporate them into recipes easily to enhance overall nutrient content.*)

In closing, I'd like to acknowledge my friend Jennifer Giles who contributed to this chapter and is responsible for not only sharing some great information, but also providing those great tips and recipe suggestions. Jenn is a Registered Dietitian / Nutritionist who specializes in Sports Dietetics. She has been in the field for over 24 years and has a unique perspective on nutrition not only as a Nutritionist but also as an athlete, a coach, the mother of 4 athletes and the wife of an athlete. Below Jenn shares her own personal story and also some interesting observations about her client's success and why she, and they, were able to find and maintain their success.

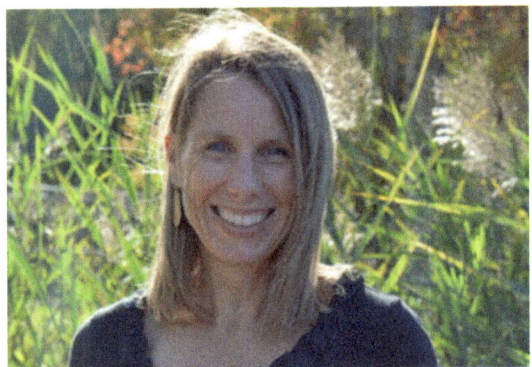

Jennifer O'Donnell-Giles, MS RD CSSD

My professional journey is deeply connected to my personal journey. I grew up in the 70s and 80s. There was never a shortage of Coke-a-Cola and Ring Dings in my house. My sideline snack during softball practice was Cool Ranch Doritos. My pre-fueling plan for swim practice was hitting up the hot dog truck (yes we had a hot dog truck pull up to our high school every day at 2:50pm). The impact of Nutrition was not on my radar, nor was it on the radar of my parents.

When I was in the 5th grade, I watched my father suffer from a heart attack. I literally watched his face turn grey, grasp his chest, and try to throw up - thinking it was a stomach virus. Then I watched out the window as my mother drove him to the Emergency Room. This happened right before Christmas. He was in the hospital for about a week. He survived. Over the next couple of months, we learned a lot about the benefits of exercising and eating well. We would take brisk walks together, eat fish, whole grains and lots of veggies. We even learned about the genetic component of heart disease.

I want to tell you that this was my eye-opening / life altering turning point. But it wasn't. I slowly fell back into old habits, grabbing those Cool Ranch Doritos again as fuel for softball. Pizza and french fries were my regular lunch order in the school cafeteria. My weight climbed and I felt sluggish and fatigued. I was not the healthy vibrant teenager I thought I should be. It is no wonder that I never realized my full athletic potential in high school. I knew I had more to give, but my team sports career ended when high school ended.

Fast forward to the summer after freshman year in college. I stopped to look at myself in the mirror and said out loud "What are you doing? Is this really how you want to live your life?" Asking myself these raw and honest questions was finally my eye-opening / life altering turning point. I purchased a pair of running shoes while on vacation that summer and set out the door to run. I hated running prior to this day so I have no idea what made me chose running. The truth is that I didn't really think about it at all. I just did it. August 18th, 1991 was the day when the trajectory of my life changed. It may have been running that was the initiation of this trajectory, but it was hands down the changes I made to my nutrition that allowed me to sustain the change for the past 31 years.

The next 3 decades since that warm August day, have included running marathons, century rides, open water swims, ironmen, and Ragnar Relays. I took the sport of running (which morphed into triathlon) to levels I never thought possible. I qualified for and completed the Boston Marathon, I competed internationally at ITU world championships. Early on, however I knew I could not keep this "new life" to myself. I was on a mission to ensure that everyone was capable of finding the joy and confidence that comes with optimal health and internal strength. I went on to obtain my degrees in nutrition and physiology and I became a dietitian. I have worked with individuals of all ages, in all sports, at all levels. The goals may be different for each person I have had the honor of working with, but the common denominator is optimal health.

I have always been curious what made me, a Ring Ding eating teenager, capable of long-term success? What makes the successful individuals that I have worked with capable of long-term success? There are plenty of people who attempt change but don't sustain it. My answer comes down to three things:

1. **Honesty.** *So many of us don't see it. Even I was blind to it. I had no idea at the time I was munching on Cool Ranch Doritos that there was a connection between the food I was putting in my body and how I was feeling or how I looked. I thought "a few chips is no big deal", after all I was eating plenty of veggies and fish and whole grains too. I assumed "It must all balance out". It was not until I*

looked in the mirror and asked myself those honest questions: "What are you doing? Is this really how you want to live your life?" was I able to admit that I was not making the right choices for my health and that I desperately needed to make a change.

2. ***Goal Setting.*** *Setting very specific goals for yourself will create a path for you to follow. Most people say, "I want to lose weight". I said the same thing initially. But it wasn't specific enough. Anyone can lose weight! That's why the diet industry is a multi-billion-dollar industry. The people who lose weight and maintain that loss have much more specific goals for themselves. Goals have to run deeper. Find your why and that will sustain you. My why was feeling good, having energy, not being tired and sluggish. If you set long term sustainable goals (vs short term weight loss goals) you will have a greater chance of achieving long term success.*

3. ***Commitment.*** *When you are being honest with yourself and setting specific long-term goals, it <u>must</u> be followed by a serious, unwavering commitment to yourself. There are necessary steps that need to be taken over and over and over again in order to achieve those goals. It's just you vs. you out there. Commit to it. Put the work in. Don't quit. Even when you reach your goals... stay on course. Trust me. You will never regret it.*

Change is at your fingertips if YOU decide you want something different from your life.

Below are 2 of my client's stories:

1. <u>From non-athlete to half ironwoman.</u>

   I'm going to call her Eliza. Eliza's husband and daughter are triathletes. Eliza was the best Sherpa and cheerleader you could have asked for. She went to every race, carried extra food, water and clothing for her husband and daughter. She would carry posters and wave pom poms and was super happy doing so.

   One day she came to me and said, "I want to try to "participate" in a race". "I don't want to race it, but I want to complete it". She was honest about wanting to transition from spectator to participant. She set a goal of entering a sprint triathlon to start with and a long-term goal of completing a half ironman. She made a commitment to her herself (along with her husband and daughter) that she was going to put the work in. Over the next few years, she put the work in. She trained regularly, sometimes alone, sometimes with friends and sometimes with her husband. She never gave up on herself even when it was really hard, when work got in the way, when it was raining, snowing, freezing cold or incredible hot and humid. She learned to fuel herself for daily training, for longer weekend sessions as well as for race day. She had many hurdles to deal with along the way including a chronic back injury and joint pain. Her specific goals and unwavering commitment to them was the reason she wasn't going to let anything stop her.

Eliza has since completed 4 sprint triathlons and 2 Olympic triathlons. She attempted her half ironman and unfortunately did not make the bike cut off time. Instead of allowing this to derail he "plan", she didn't allow herself to consider this a failure. She immediately signed up for another one two months later and on that day SHE DID IT!!

She continues to train and "participate" to this day.

Take away: *Your journey will look different than everyone else's. It's supposed to! It's unique to you, your goals and your capabilities. Create change based on what you want to accomplish and how you want to tell your life story when you look back.*

2. It's never too late.

   I'm going to call him Charlie. Charlie came to me at the age of 47. He had a wife, 3 teenage children and a very stressful 80 per hour week job. He had not worked out in over a decade and ate out every day. He would skip breakfast due to his long commute, grab a granola bar for lunch and eat out at restaurants for work dinners 3-4 times a week. He also traveled ALOT, so convenient grab and go food was how he described his diet. The first time I met Charlie he said, "I need you to help me lose 50 pounds".

   Charlie was a Division 1 college lacrosse player. So, his initial goal was to get back to "college weight". When we dug a little deeper, I learned that his diet was always focused on convenient grab and go food. Charlie never learned how to eat. I love using Charlie as an example. Most of us were never taught how to eat. Sure our parents told us to eat our fruits and veggies. But we never learned the true science behind how nutrients are responsible for our cell turnover. How fiber strengthens our gut microbiome and improves immunity. How hydration helps lessen the workload of our hearts. And so much more…

   Once Charlie learned the science behind what food does for us, his mindset changed completely. He began moving his body again slowly and found a love for hiking. He worked his way from a 1 mile hike to a 12 mile hike in the Adirondacks within 12 months. He went from grabbing a donut and coffee for a snack to munching on trail mix and unsweetened iced tea to get him through busy work afternoons. What I found most profound about Charlie, was that he focused on fueling his body. His goal went from wanting to lose 50 pounds, to fueling his body in order to have more energy each day, feel happier and be able to get his hike in almost every day of the week. Yes the weight came off - but only after he learned how to eat and fueled his body optimally. He now can say that he feels better at 50 years old than he did playing lax in college.

Take away: *If you change your mindset and you will change your life. Sometimes what you think is the answer is not the correct answer. Weight loss is the goal for so many. It was for me initially! I get that! But in order to have a long-term sustainable goal there has to be more. You must have goals that are directly connected to feeling good and truly being healthy. Feeling amazing IS your motivation for long term success.*

You can find out more about Jenn and reach out to her on Instagram and TikTok @jenngileseat4sport, on Facebook: @ THE SPORTS NUTRITION HUB and on LinkedIn @ Jennifer O'Donnell-Giles.

For many people, creating successful nutrition strategies will be the hardest part of their wellness plan. We've shared a lot of information in this chapter, but don't jump into every area at once. Begin to modify your nutritional habits slowly and remember we aren't pushing a diet; we are trying to change habits to allow for a lifetime of healthy living. Let's try to identify and frame food for its primary purpose, to fuel the body. When we eat the right types of foods, in the right quantities, we feel better and have the energy necessary to have our body work for us. Remember that there is no perfect diet and while it doesn't sound exciting: fruits, vegetables and lean proteins are what your body needs. Don't forget how the thermic effect of food can be used to increase your metabolism and that this strategy is even more effective with frequent smaller meals. Lastly, remember not to compare yourselves to others and to focus on controlling what you can.

Nutritional Guidelines

Eat Every 2-3 Hours
Have a goal of 5-8 smaller meals per day. Remember the thermic effect of food and how it can increase your metabolism by up to 20% based on the foods you consume.

Eat Complete Meals
Focus on lean proteins and having either a fruit or vegetable with each meal.

Eat Complex Carbohydrates
Focus on whole grain rice, fruits, and vegetables. Remember simple (sugars) carbohydrates are what lead to weight gain.

Eat Good Fats
Ensure that 25-35% of your energy intake comes from fat, primarily from monounsaturated (e.g., olive oil) and polyunsaturated (e.g., flax oil, salmon oil). Remember "good" fats will not make you fat. Healthy fats provide a multitude of health benefits.

Avoid Sugar and Fat Free Foods
Free normally means more sugar or chemical sugar substitutes. Neither is good for your body.

Eat Whole Foods
Avoid processed foods and try to eat things in their whole state. Examples are whole fruits and vegetables coupled with lean proteins. Avoid processed foods especially sugars and trans fats.

Drink Water
Drink 6-8 cups of water a day and focus on healthy choices like green tea and avoid drinks high in sugar.

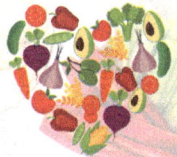
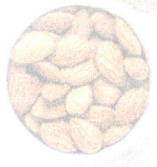

Chapter 7:
Your Crucible

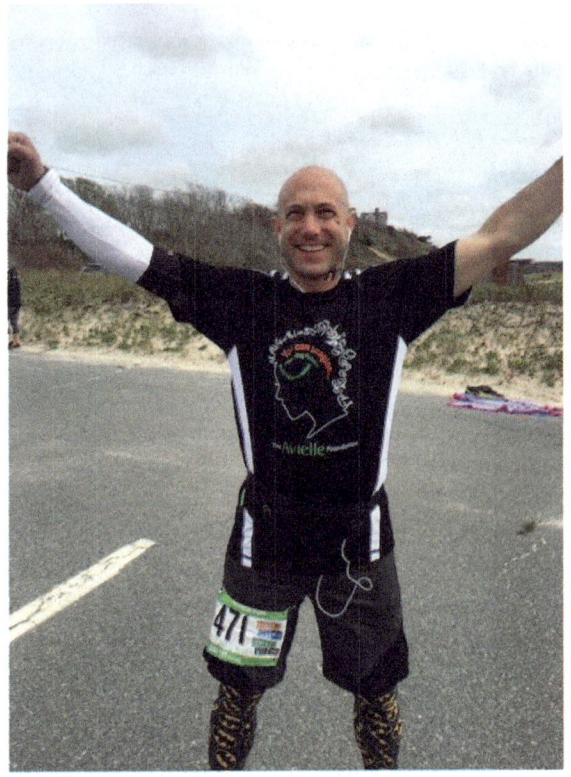

"The most beautiful people I've known are those who have known trials, have known struggles, have known loss, and have found their way out of the depths." – Elizabeth Kübler-Ross

Nothing in life worth talking about ever happens in your comfort zone. Embarking on a healthier lifestyle will create physical challenges that will require discipline and sacrifice. However, you will find that there is another level in all of us that will surface during extreme circumstances when you are forced to deal with adversity. **This is your crucible.**

To this point, we have discussed goals based on improving baseline metrics and building a functional body that will allow you to live your best life. We have, in a very controlled manner, followed a progression to develop good habits to ensure success. Well, now it's time to break away from numbers and guidelines and test your new body and your will as we enter the crucible phase of The Method. Your crucible will re-sharpen your focus and rejuvenate your motivation. For any of you that have ever played sports, we are tapping into that competitive drive. If you have never played a sport, think of the fear and doubt that became exhilaration when you overcame an obstacle, like public speaking. So for your crucible, I want you to create a physical goal for yourself even if you aren't sure if you can do it!

The sky's the limit and this expectation is being driven by you. You will need to choose something that will focus your efforts, fears, and greatest internal motivators so that when you are done, you will feel a tremendous sense of pride in the process you took to prepare for your goal. Maybe it's running your first 5k or participating in a Tough Mudder (an endurance event series where participants attempt 10-to-12-mile-long obstacle courses) or a TriAthlon. As long as the process of planning and preparing for the event will push you to work harder than you think you can, it will qualify as a crucible. It's possible that you may not be able to accomplish your goal right away, but the process will put you on another journey of self-discovery that will further boost your confidence in your ability to transform. The memories formed as you try to accomplish what was previously considered impossible will instill you with a lifetime of memories and confidence. "Shoot for the stars. You may not get the stars – but you may get the moon." -Carleton Young

The term crucible event comes from a friend, the late Dr. Jeremy Richman. As a neuroscientist, he demonstrated the tremendous benefits to the brain, psyche, and soul that this type of goal setting can have on individuals. He was a huge believer in crucible challenges. Jeremy and his wife started the Avielle Foundation in honor of their daughter to advance our understanding of the brain and to prevent violence. The Avielle Foundations legacy of building compassion and reducing violence continues under The Avielle Initiative, which operates as a program within the National Mental Health Innovation Center (NMHIC). I encourage you to visit their website at www.cuanschutz.edu.

For me personally, I love this type of challenge and have engaged in many crucible events. However, the one which is most dear to my heart takes place in my community each December. Now termed the Crucible Challenge, this unique event involves a group of us running either a 5 mile or a ½ marathon course followed by a jump into the freezing cold waters of a local lake. The physical and emotional toll of accomplishing the run is nothing compared to the overwhelming weight of the freezing cold water as you submerge your body into it. This event is so special because *it's underground and authentic in every way possible!* There is no fee, no clock, no sponsor, no fundraising, no uniform, no course markers associated with this event. Our only goal is to finish and connect with some great people along the way.

Finishing and connecting is such an important part of this event that we've created a tradition termed "The Return Loop". We encourage every runner as they finish to turn back or loop back onto the course to pick up any runners that are still on the course to encourage them to finish. So just think about this notion for a minute, usually once someone finishes a race the mind and body both immediately disengage from the strenuous activity and a sense of relief, accomplishment and pride sets in. However, during the Crucible Challenge, you personally finish but then immediately head back onto the course to run side by side with others as they too reach the finish. Adding to that physical and mental challenge is the fact that the last few hundred yards of the race is a significant downhill (with the beautiful lake in the background). But in keeping with the theme of the day, our 'tribe' of runners finish the run together before plunging into the cold and perhaps icy (!) lake.

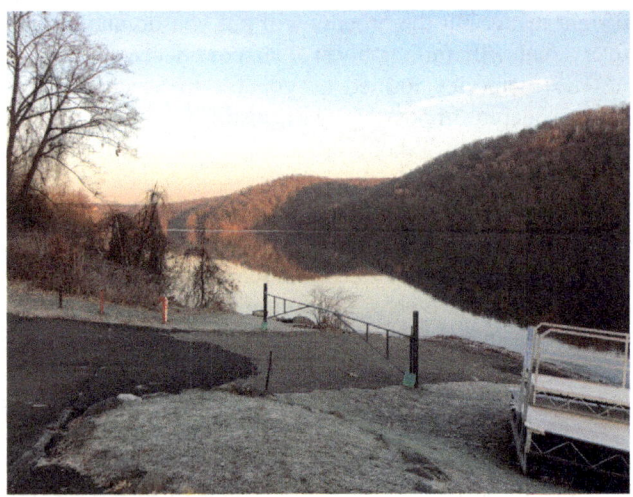

The inspiration experienced by both the active runners as well as those coming back onto the course is magical. Science has demonstrated acts of kindness benefit both the recipient as well as the giver. Additionally, anyone that observes acts of kindness will also be positively impacted. So "The Return Loop" literally inspires and connects everyone that comes in contact with it. Clearly not an easy task, particularly as some folks have already run a ½ marathon, but for me this tradition speaks to every level of a crucible event and the power of connection.

Another example of a Crucible Event comes from a friend of mine, Nick Waaler. Nick is a guy with a huge heart that would do anything to help a friend and his story is truly amazing and personifies a crucible challenge.

More importantly, his journey to achieving his crucible speaks volumes to how anyone of us can do something amazing with the right mindset, support, motivation and determination.

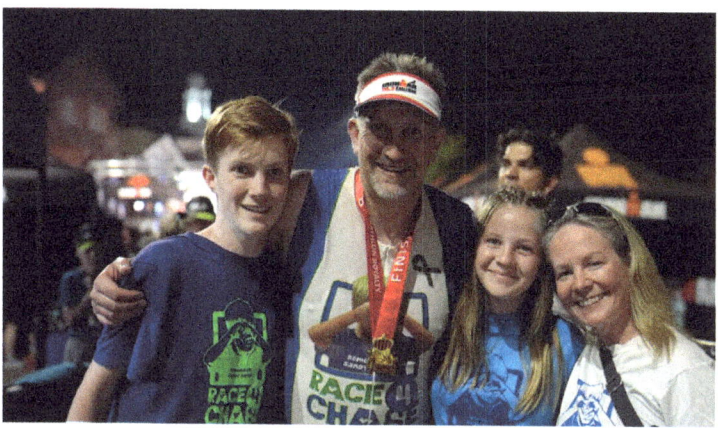

Below is Nick's story...

I was never a runner back in 2012 - I never understood why people ran for fun - this was a foreign concept for me. Only time I ever ran was if I had a ball and someone else wanted it or the other way round. In 2013 Ian Hockley (COINCIDENTALLY, IAN IS REFERNCED IN THIS BOOK SEVEAL DIFFERN'T TIMES) asked me if I ran, and after laughing that off thinking the crazy man had finished, he then asked me the question that changed my life in an incredible way. Funnily enough it had nothing to do with running. He asked me "Well, can you drive then?" Damn this man, he knows I can drive, why is he asking, is this a trick question ? So I answered hesitantly that "Yes I can drive". "Great, you are now a driver for a Ragnar team" What ?!?!?! What is Ragnar ??!!?!?

For those of you who aren't sure what a Ragnar Race is – it's a 200ish mile relay race, run in teams of 12 or teams of 6 if you are an ultra runner. It starts on a Friday morning and generally finishes Saturday afternoon. Each runner runs 3 legs of approx. 3 to 10 miles each leg. So at this meeting there were Ragnarians who had run it in 2013, now maybe it was the video of their experience, or maybe it was the cool Ragnar attire they were wearing, maybe it was the inspirational talk given by Ian, OR maybe it was the beer that gave me some extra bravado, but I was inspired, I turned to Ian and said I can do this, I can run, sign me up, find another driver.

Out came the app "Couch to 5k" and my new running life started ! I have since completed 6 regular Ragnars up in Cape Cod and one Ultra Ragnar in Hamburg, Germany. About a year after I started running, I saw a picture of Chase Kowalski, age 6, holding his medal after completing and winning his one and only triathlon and something inside me was moved to think that this was my calling. I was deeply touched by his story, teaching himself, asking his parents to enter him into a race - I mean WOW !! At the time I was barely aware of triathlons let alone that kids did them too, and here was Chase owning it.

Well, if he was able to do this, then I too, wanted to start and see what it was all about. Over the next 4 years, I trained and completed the different stages of the triathlon world starting with the Sprint Tris, moving on up to the Olympic Tris, then in 2019 I did my first Half Ironman and once that was in the bag I felt ready to take on a full 140.6 Ironman - so I signed up for Ironman Lake Placid 2020, known to be one of the toughest Ironman courses globally.

Well, we all know that Covid struck and shut down the world, devastating so many lives. Obviously Lake Placid 2020 was then cancelled and not wanting to waste all my training I told Rebecca Kowalski that I wanted to do my own Ironman here in Sandy Hook itself. Rebecca came up with the name Iron "Chase".

So in September 2020 I completed an Ironman on my own, it was simply an epic event, with friends and family all being a part of it, either supporting, biking sections with me or running parts of the marathon with me, culminating two passes of Chase's bench in Wolfe Park and ending at Chase's family home. We raised over $15,000 that day.

Now going back to when I was training for my Sprint Tri - doing my 10 laps - I would imagine what it must be like to finish a full Ironman, it was a dream well above my station, but I thought about how amazing it would be - well that finish at Chase's house was even more incredible than I could ever have imagined with all my friends and family there and Chase's family - I had my own personal finish line !!

Well, I completed an Ironman distance - would I do it again. The plan wasn't to do another one, the amount of training and time away from the family, it was suggested that this should not happen !! But.....I had this deferral in my pocket and I still wanted to do an "official" Ironman - I really wanted to do this for Chase. I got the all clear and so the training all started again and we managed to get to the start line which is the reward for all the training - the hardest part of an Ironman is getting to the start line injury free.
So here we were at the start line of Lake Placid - five years in the making from non runner to starting my second full Ironman - my first "official" one. This is how it went down....

The Swim

By the time, my friend Liz and I had gotten down to the lake front for the swim start, the pros had already started - we heard the start cannon go off on the two minute walk to the start. The start is self graded and I lined up in the 1hr 30 to 1hr 45 section - hoping to finish before 1hr 45mins which was the time I swam when I did it in the pool for the Iron"Chase" back in September. To begin with Liz was also lined up with me which I thought was odd as she is a really good swimmer but she said she didn't want to go all out - so I didn't say anything. Then she realized that the times posted were not pace times but estimated finish times so we hugged it out - wished each other the best and we will meet again at the finish - Liz then moved up to where she should be starting !!

While waiting, the announcer was introducing certain athletes such as the oldest competitor, a 71 year old woman and then the youngest who was 18 years old and was enlisting into the Army the next day - both of whom got big cheers and applause. So my time to start came and I was in the water at 653am - I looked into the crowd one last time to see if I could see my family and give them a wave but not sure where they were - so jumped in knowing I would see them soon enough at the beginning of the bike ride. The first half mile or so of the swim did not go too well as I was unable to get into my swimming rhythm - I couldn't put my head in the water and do my regular swim strokes / breathing and I had to swim with my head out of the water - this has happened before in my open water swims and it's open water anxiety that I have no control over - I'm mentally fine and not concerned but my brain and body are just not adapting - as I said I wasn't concerned as it's just a matter of time before I'm fine and can start swimming normally and swim like I'm in the pool.

That moment came around the half mile mark - half way through lap 1. I swam the second half just fine with a little off course swimming due to poor sighting. After one loop, I was back at the start, where you get out of the water for a few seconds as you loop through the timing mat and jump back in for the second half.

A little knowledge about the Lake Placid swim - this is a famous swim as there is a cable about 3 feet underwater that connects all the buoys and if you can follow that cable you firstly have the most direct route and secondly you don't have to sight. There is no issue losing sight of the cable once you see it as the water is crystal clear. However with that advantage comes with the fact that pretty much everyone wants to be near it, and if you don't like crowded swimming with people all over you it might not be the place to be ! I did not want any of that so on the first lap I kept to the left of the crowd and relied on my sighting of the buoys.

With all that being said, when I jumped in for the second loop I started swimming and noticed this cord/line below me and realized I was swimming with the cable and no-one was around me. I owned that cable for the rest of my swim and swam my best open water swim finishing in 1hr 26mins - nearly 20mins faster than my Iron"Chase" pool swim !! I was a little annoyed as I could have been quicker were it not for my slow half mile at the beginning. Either way I was pumped !!

The Bike

Jumped on the bike and started out - passed, my friend, Cathy and her family at beginning of bike ride, rode through town, gave huge waves as I passed Neasa, Aidan and Teagan and Liz's family at mile 2 - now I was on my own. Me and my thoughts for next 8 hours ! Was already looking forward to getting to pass the family for the second time but there was a long way to go before that. Rode the ascent out of Placid and remembered that Mark Russell was going to be at the Aid Station by the Bob Sled Stadium. The trick about doing triathlons is to break it up in sections - buoy to buoy on the swim, 10 mile marker to 10 mile marker on the bike and mile to mile on the run.

There was a huge descent into Keene which I was a little nervous about as the roads were still very slick and there were cross winds and on coming traffic - obviously our side of the road was closed to traffic but still I was about to go down a mountain for about 5-7 miles at about 35-40 mph. It was exhilarating and scary at the same time, knowing that one mistake will be the end of the race and most likely a trip to the hospital. On both laps I passed an ambulance and a rider being tended to on this descent and later found out that there had been a couple of nasty accidents.

So I made it to Keene and enjoyed the ride to mile 35 where there is a 5 mile out and back and you get to see all the other riders ahead of you for a little while.

So carried on until the North Pole which is where we turned left back to Lake Placid - 12 miles to go until halfway. This is the ascent, where we climb Baby Bear, Momma Bear and Poppa Bear and it was tough, hard and brutal and worst of all, it's in your head that you have to come back and this will be your last 10 miles before transition. Not only that we had to fight a full on headwind right in our face !! Baby Bear and Momma Bear were long gradual uphills and I won't forget seeing Poppa Bear - it looks so different on a bike than in a car ! I turned the corner having come onto a little flat after completing Baby and Momma Bears and then you see Poppa Bear, not a long hill but the incline looked like a mountain - you could see the *start and end and the crowds on it cheering everyone ahead of you and the music blaring - this was going to be a battle.*

I cursed it out but made it to the top - it was now a quick ride into town and back the way I came and then into transition area to refill my water and my nutrition.

About 70 miles in I was also starting to suffer from "hot feet" - Hot feet is a common malady on rides that last 3 hours or more, so it affects century riders, tourers and cyclists who just like to go long. The primary cause is the tendency of feet to swell during long rides. This increases pressure inside the shoes, which, in turn, compresses nerves which starts a set of symptoms in which the feet often become uncomfortably hot and painful.. Over the next 30 or so miles I needed to stop a couple of times to take off my cycling shoes and stretch out and cool down my feet - this always seems to work and I do feel better after doing this.

Anyway I reach mile 104 and passing through an Aid Station and there seems to be more cyclists here than the usual amount and the atmosphere seems a little different. I keep riding as wasn't planning on stopping as there were only 8 miles left and I had to be out of transition by 530pm and it was just past 430pm. As I was coming to the end of the Aid Station there was a man in the middle of the road with some cyclists around him with his hand up in the air telling me to stop - this was odd - I slowed down and came to a stop, wondering what was happening. He said that "you have missed the cut off - you race ends here" !!!!

I was in shock, it had not entered my mind that I would miss any of the cut offs on the course - so much stuff was going thru my head about letting my family down, letting Chase and his family down, how disappointed all my friends would be, what about the BCC live crew who were also waiting/wanting me to finish - this didn't make any sense to me !?!

There was this one guy on a regular bike on the other side of the road that was disputing everything too - I don't know who he was but he seemed to know the rules but wasn't an official - he wasn't a competitor either and I have no idea why he happened to be there but he was sowing doubt into my mind and a few others over the veracity of this cut off. It got to the point that a few of us just decided to continue on with the race despite what this official was saying - he said if we continued we would be disqualified but at this point what did it matter between a DQ and DNF (did not finish).

I heard him note my number as I passed him, but told myself he had to get everyone's number - he couldn't just DQ me. Either way I was now pumped to finish as quickly as possible - and these last 8 miles were all uphill remember. I was worried that I was going to get pulled over any minute by an official on a motorbike or that I would be pulled over by the penalty tent that I had to pass later. I'm cycling much faster up these last hills than the first lap - all this time this stranger is cycling with us on the other side of the road - he's just encouraging us to keep going and that this will be sorted - who was this man ??

I came into Transition in a world of mental battles - I was rushed - I didn't want to be rushed out of transition. I was spent - I had just pounded that last 8 miles uphill to get here as quick as possible. I had been told my race was over. I had also been told that everything was fine. The last 40 or so minutes I had been worried that someone was going to pull me over and stop me.

Oh and there was also the fact that part of my brain was gleeful that my race was over because that meant I didn't have to run the marathon part - I was fighting myself too!! I opened my run bag and for some reason my sneakers were soaking wet - so wet that I poured water out of them. How ???? What can I do - can't worry about that - just put them on - at least my socks are dry (they were in a Ziplock). Put all my bike gear in my now empty run bag. Put on my Camelback and headed out towards the Run Out chute. All these things going thru my head over the course of 7 minutes of transition.

The Run

I leave transition and again no one has stopped me - I'm now assuming I'm good to go but mentally I am still not ready. I ask someone in the crowd what time it was just so I have a base time of when I started the run, this turned out to be huge, more on that later. At this point, I'm walking, trying to eat a sandwich, and all I'm thinking is that there is no way I have the time or the energy left in me to complete a marathon and then I realized I also forgot to grab my salt tabs out of my bike bag during my rushed transition. Shit !

Mentally I was probably in my worst place the whole race - before the race you know you will hit those negative mental blocks and you think you will be ready for them but when they come it is a real battle to keep going. This is when you need to feed off the vibe of all the support around you.

I bumped into Cathy and her family again at the first aid station and I told her about my salt situation and she told me not to worry and that she had some at her rental and would head back and get some and get on her bike and catch up and give to me at the next aid station - this was a positive.

It was at the five mile mark where things took a turn for the better - I looked at my watch and saw that I had completed 5 miles in 1hr 05mins - which wasn't too bad. It gave me a boost to start doing some math to see if I could indeed get to the finish on time. When did I start the run - yes, I asked someone, what was it ? 5.20pm. Ok. I have until midnight. That gives me 6hrs 40mins. That should be plenty of time. Let's break this marathon down. I have 3hrs 20mins to get to 13 miles and 1hr 40mins for each 6.5 mile section. Ok. Ok. Let's see where we are at when I get to 6.5 miles. I kept going and reached the 6.5 mile point at 1hr 28mins. Ok Ok - this is great - I just bought myself 12 minutes - this is huge. This was the moment when I actually realized I could possibly finish. If I maintained this pace for the next 19.5 miles I could finish, barring any cramping, or my body shutting down and that I have enough nutrition to get to the finish.

I was starving hungry at this point but didn't have enough energy to wolf down an energy bar so over the next hour I was breaking off tiny pieces of it and eating it bit by bit. My next goal was to get to the 13 mile point within 3hrs 20mins - if I did that - then the last cut off at 9pm at the 13.5 mile marker would not come into play and then all I had to do would be to get to the finish before midnight. They were starting to light all the floodlights on River Road as there are no street lights and it was starting to get late now ! I got to the 13 mile point and ran to it with Teagan, which was great, and I was in much better spirits when I saw Neasa and Aidan this time around. I made it in 03hrs 03mins - I had just bought myself another five minutes and now had seventeen minutes in credit - this was very encouraging and the cramp onsets were happening less and less frequently.

I made the turnaround and headed out for my second lap and my next goal was to get to the 19.5 mile point within 5hrs. I passed Neasa and the kids one more time knowing this was the last time I would see them before the finish line.

I was maintaining a steady pace now, walking up the little hills and through the aid stations where I would drink water or coke and eat the chips or pretzels whenever necessary and soon there would be chicken broth at some of the aid stations and I was looking forward to that. The second biggest moment of the day came at mile 19.5 when I got there at 4hrs 42mins and realized I had a little under 2hrs to get to the finish line. I knew at this moment that I was ACTUALLY going to finish - I had run all three of my 6.5 mile sections in under 1hr 40mins and there was no way that I was going to take more than two hours to run this last 6.5 miles. I was now pumped, I had won the mental fight - let's get this over !!

I turned and Cathy told me that my family was at the finish line waiting for me and to go finish like an Ironman !

I started running, passing a couple of other soon to be Ironman's, reached the finish chute, which was still packed with supporters all cheering and banging their hands on the chute, the fireworks went off and I heard Mike Reilly "the voice of Ironman" calling my name and telling me that I was an "Ironman" and there was Neasa, Aidan and Teagan all waiting for me, Neasa medaled me and I just embraced them all - I had achieved my goal that I had dreamed about 6 years earlier. Even though I was wrecked I felt on top of the world and was able to share that moment with the most important people in my life !

So, what will your crucible be? I'd suggest you start spending some time now and dream big! You can continue to develop your goal while embarking on your fitness journey and may become more inspired as you become more fit. Remember that it's the journey or the process of accomplishing your crucible that will change your life as much as actually accomplishing the crucible itself. Your journey, whether you know it or not, could be starting as you read this chapter and map out your steps to becoming more fit.

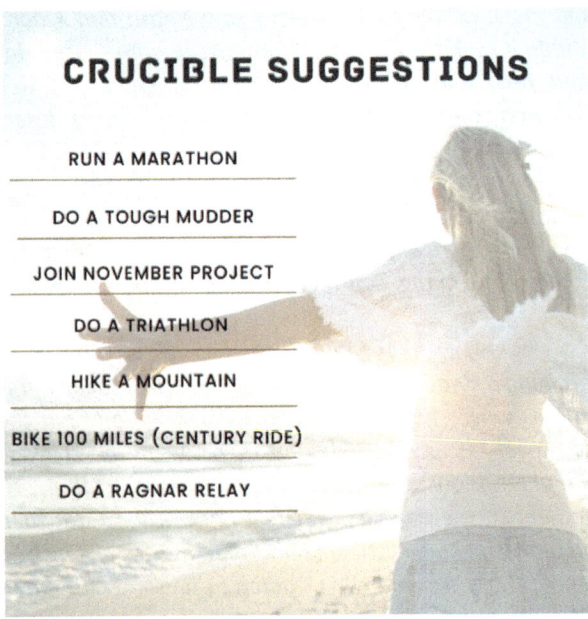

Chapter 8:
Connect with Others to Inspire their Journey

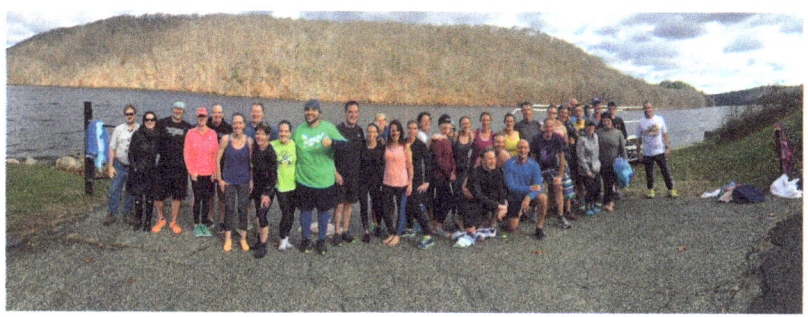

"It's about Love, Connection and Being Human"
As humans, we are wired to connect with each other. Whether you are an introvert or an extrovert, the power of connecting with each other is vital to the human experience. As discussed earlier, when coupled with a crucible challenge this process can forge relationships and further enhance the experience. Scientists have supported that when we find groups or connect with others we can manage stress better and live more fulfilling lives. We know that exercise and nutrition improve just about every physical, emotional, and mental condition known to man. When you combine these physical benefits with the opportunity to develop as a human being, you have to ask, what are you waiting for? If there were a pill that promised to make you feel happier, sleep better, have more energy, have less stress, live longer, and accomplish physical goals, would you take it? You sure would, as would I. Well, the blueprint for a better life can start with improving your health and incorporating and connecting with others as part of that process.

Transformation is very powerful. I have spent most of my career on the "front lines" of the battle against weight gain. Countless times I have witnessed the overwhelming sense of accomplishment, pride, and joy of watching people accomplish their goals. However, what has been more moving than observing their individual successes has been observing the ripple effect. When a parent can inspire their children, or a co-worker can motivate their peers, we begin to see a true community impact take place. One of the proudest experiences of my career has been watching successful clients of mine become trainers themselves. Their personal success led to a contagious spirit. They wanted to share how good they felt about themselves and in turn, help others change their lives. It's beyond measure to feel connected to someone transforming themselves, but you don't need to be a trainer to provide support.

This past summer a friend of mine invited a few of us to swim at his lake house. The house is situated on a quiet and peaceful lake that doesn't allow motorized crafts. He had recently bought the place and wanted to start swimming for exercise. On the first day a few of us met, we made it across the lake and back one time and absolutely loved the experience. Before long more people joined our group and we were consistently meeting every Wednesday and Sunday morning for a 6am swim. In summers past, I swam laps at the town pool when I had time or felt like it. But very quickly I found myself adjusting my calendar around meeting this group for our 6am swim. This group and these swims became my priority, we were all counting on each other to be there. By the end of the summer, my friend was in significantly better shape, we were all swimming across the lake and back twice at a clip and felt great about ourselves and the experience.

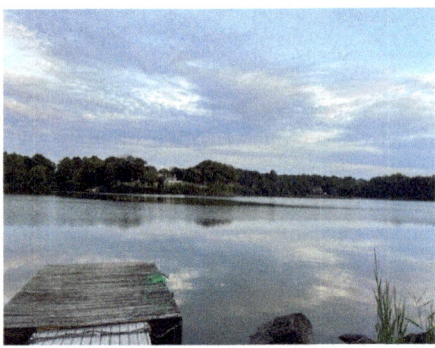

Ironically one morning, one of our members, Bob, told me about this amazing nonprofit out of Boston called the November Project. He was sharing how the organization formed, which was actually very similar to our little swim group. Two guys made a pact to meet every day at 6:30am during the month of November to workout together. Since that original promise, those two guys, Brogan Graham and Bojan Mandaric, ignited a social fitness phenomenon called the November Project.

The November Project (NP) has since grown to hundreds of members who exercise multiple times a week in a number of cities around the United States, Canada, Asia and Europe. These free workouts are all led by volunteers, most of whom were at one point members themselves. Inspired by their work, I connected with and was fortunate enough to sit down and talk to one of the founders, Bojan Mandaric, to learn how two guys were able to positively impact so many lives. My conversation was informative, inspirational and also validating as it was quickly evident that Bojan shared similar beliefs in the power of human connection and experienced firsthand the impact it can have on wellness.

Bojan began by describing the immense satisfaction and surprise at how his pact with one led from one person showing up to join them on the first day to ultimately hundreds joining them for what is now one of their signature Harvard Stadium workouts. He then described what he now believes are the key factors to that many people showing up for these workouts, regardless of weather or other challenges. For those of you familiar with the Northeast in the Winter, outdoor workouts can prove brutal! Just showing up might be one of the most important elements of their success. This group is about inclusion and regardless of your level of fitness, there is a sense that if you can just show up, you have already succeeded.

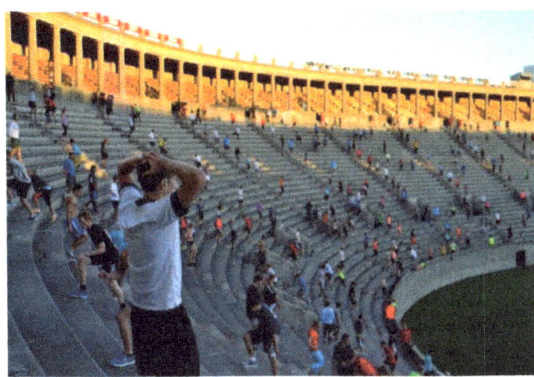
November Project Harvard Stadium Workout

The November Project focuses on simple but powerful messaging that we can all relate to. "Beating the alarm clock" is their expression that represents the internal fight one has on a cold morning where staying in bed with a comfortable pillow and a warm blanket is much more appealing than going outside into the cold for a workout. Outside of relying on one's personal motivation, NP employs a strategy called "Accountability Buddies" to help get folks to "beat the alarm clock". These Accountability Buddies are the individual or individuals who have committed to meet each other. NP uses a simple term, a "Verbal" which suggests that your "word is your bond" and if I'm telling you I will be there, then I will be there. This simple agreement provides accountability to yourself and to the person you are supposed to meet. I think we can all agree with Bojan when he said that "It's so much easier to go through something challenging if you have someone alongside of you than if you have to go through it by yourself".

For me, this is both powerful and again validating as I have experienced this type of relationship and commitment so many times in my life. Whether in sports, training, or community programs, somewhere along the way, there was always an Accountability Buddy for me. If you haven't experienced this yet, I strongly urge you to try and let's all use the unquestionable success of the November Project as the measure of success to validate this power.

Bojan also shared that he's witnessed social connections grow outside of just the workouts. Members gather together to create smaller niche groups for both social events and to connect on other fitness interests. I've also experienced this firsthand and so many of the relationships I have in my life were formed through wellness initiatives I either created or participated in.

Lastly, Bojan shared a powerful message about making workouts fun and even incorporating a level of silliness. I appreciate this message as we often experience levels of mental, physical and emotional fatigue with working out, regardless of how well the program has been designed. I covered this earlier in the book, although I didn't go so far as to use the word "silly", but this aligns very much with Steve Gross and the Life is Good Playmakers philosophy. Steve Gross talked about the power of Optimism, which is built on many variables and includes "Fun". So, if two leaders in the world of fitness and human connection believe that fun and silliness can help us connect, then let's listen to them and incorporate a little more fun into our workouts! Let's bring back the spirit of our youth to play and not just work out. We can still deliver the same outcome but enjoy the process more and probably add a little more balance to our lives as well.

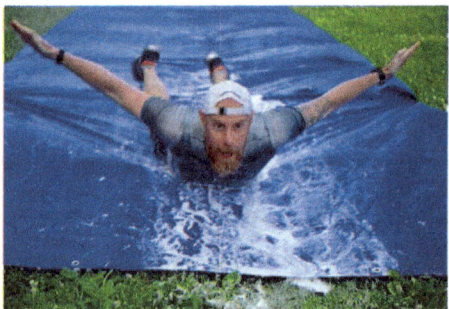

Co-Founder and Executive Director at November Project.

For more information on The November Project please visit https://november-project.com/.

It's hard to measure the power of connection scientifically, but when an organization like November Project has accomplished so much success built on human connection and accountability, it really validates for me that "Connection" is indeed one of the most powerful tools we have to sustain a healthy wellness lifestyle.

When I think of the power of connection, I can't not think of my friend Ian Hockley. Ian is a true inspiration. He's reminiscent of the "ordinary" superhero like Superman/ Spiderman in that he appears unassuming in his day-to-day life until he's called into action and the costume comes on. Ian's costume may only be a mere pair of sneakers when inspiring thousands of people to run or maybe a hoodie when he's passionately presenting about his amazing nonprofit Dylan's Wing of Change, but his impact is unmeasurable. Anybody that's ever been around him, heard his story, and seen his desire to connect people, instantly becomes inspired to want to do more, be better and help someone else. While Ian's journey may have been fueled by grief, he has since inspired thousands of people through the power of connection and has honored his son with an amazing legacy. From countless engagements on a local level to being a nationally recognized speaker and co-founder and executive director of the not-for-profit, Dylan's Wings of Change, Ian Hockley is making a difference.

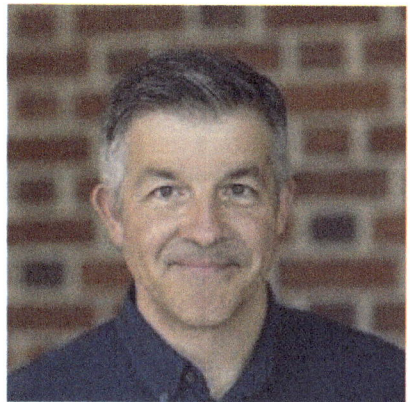

Co-Founder and Executive Director of Dylan's Wings of Change.

Below is Ian's story...

When I moved to Sandy Hook, Connecticut in 2011 I had just turned 40 and was 20lbs overweight, never finding the time to work out between career and young family commitments. Energized by the faster pace of life in the US, I returned to the Karate training that I had left off in my youth and started running that year to get in better shape. After a couple of 5K races I decided to commit to running the Manhattan half marathon in January 2013. Like so many in the community I had joined, my world changed completely on December 14, 2012 when my youngest son Dylan was one of the 20 1st-graders killed in the Sandy Hook Elementary mass school alongside six of their brave educators. Through the stupor of grief I ran that half in Central Park, finding some relief in the challenge of what was the longest distance I had ever attempted.

My friends at the Karate club wanted to raise money for the fledgling foundation we had created for Dylan's memory. One of them had heard about a crazy 200 mile relay race, running day and night. Without any real understanding of what we were in for, we formed a team of 12 runners and two drivers for our transport vans and entered "Dylan's Wings of Change" in the Cape Cod Ragnar Relay in May of 2013. We spent 3 months researching, planning and training. In that 48 hours of constant companionship, on the road and in the vans, we found ourselves again. There were tears a-plenty, but equally joyous as much as from sorrow. In the low moments we picked each other up and forged ahead. We didn't care how long it took, we were going to finish the race as a team.

We named Dylan's foundation after that first team, and over the years have recruited over 400 people on dozens of teams to run Ragnar's in three countries. At our peak in 2015 there were more than 100 of us gathered at the start line, wearing our purple shirts emblazoned "Running for Dylan". Some of the other foundations dedicated to Sandy Hook victims began entering teams in the same race. It became both a huge family and a massive party, no-one was bothered about "winning", and every time that feeling of togetherness and why we were there got us through.

My passion for this race series got me noticed by Ragnar and I joined their ranks of Ambassadors - unpaid fanatics who spread the word wherever they go. Through travels to their offices in Utah and Reebok's HQ in Mass., I met ultra-runners for the first time, that's anything above a marathon distance. A whole new world was opened up to me, and in recent years I have run two 50-milers and attempted two 100 milers. And while I did not finish either of the latter, I came to realize the real success was that I managed to run 62 miles in both of them. When we set our goals far beyond what we believe we can do, we will be amazed about what we are really capable of.

It has been fascinating to watch the journey of those that have joined us on these adventures. My friend Nick came to an early Ragnar recruitment evening back in 2014. "Sorry Ian, I came along to support you, but I only run to tackle a guy carrying a ball". I asked if he could drive a van, to which he could only say yes. One of their team dropped out and Nick was elevated to running three legs of the relay. He returned the next year and ran further than before. A couple of years later he entered his first triathlon, and the tables turned and he recruited a few of us to join him in the water, on the bike and running the road. He joined us in Germany where 5 of us ran 170 miles in one of the first Ragnar's in Europe. Nick then took the ultimate challenge and entered the Lake Placid Ironman, and when it was cancelled by the COVID-19 lockdown, he completed the distance he had trained for in his hometown. He continued to train and when the race returned in 2021 he crossed the finish line and heard those life changing words "Nick Waaler, you are AN IRONMAN!" Nick is an example of that virtuous circle where he now inspires me to try harder and go further.

The power of this camaraderie is none more evident than in our Wingman *program. We work with groups of kids or adults and through experiential learning based activities help them forge genuine connections and natural bonds. These established relationships create support networks that help stem the tide of an increasingly disconnected society. Our trained leaders and mentors then go out and work in their community, spreading their new found positivity like ripples in a pond.*

At Dylan's Wings of Change we believe in the Butterfly Effect, that small changes will accumulate building to a massive impact. The butterfly flapping its wings can cause a hurricane. That when a good deed is done and passed on, the effects are limitless. Every person you inspire to make change continues that ripple.

So, while we can't all be the next Ian Hockley, we can make a difference in at least one person's life. Fitness, like kindness, is contagious. We can grow both and be the change that creates healthier, happier more fulfilling lives. So, as you embark on your fitness journey I challenge you to make a difference in someone else's life as well – Find a way to help at least one person along their fitness journey.

For more information on Ian's organization, Dylan's Wings of Change, please visit https://www.dylanswingsofchange.org/.

Connect...

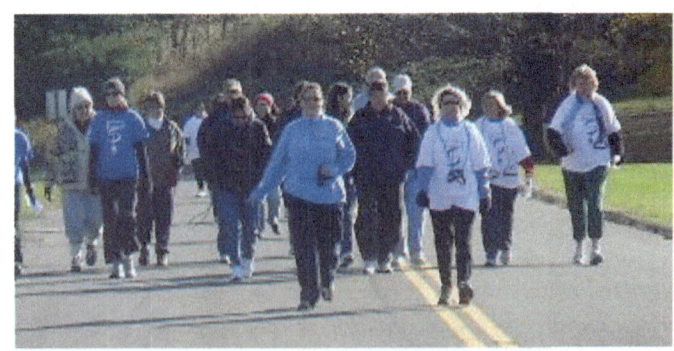
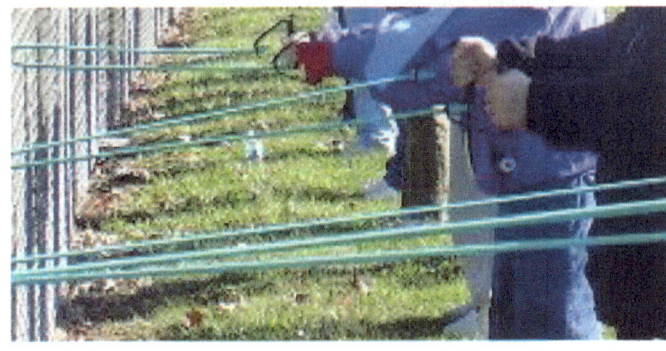
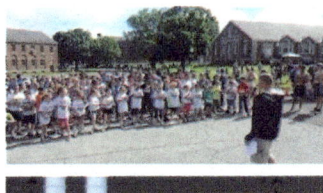
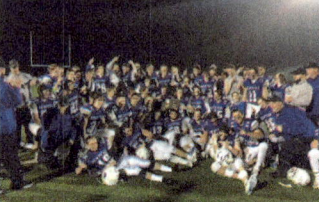
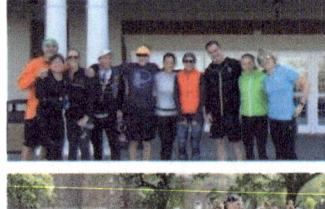
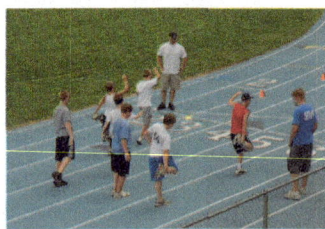
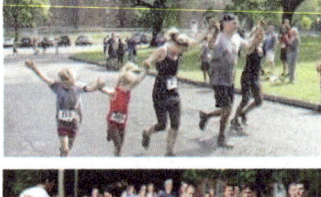
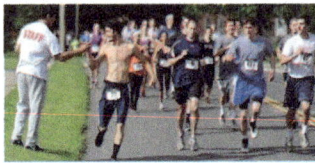
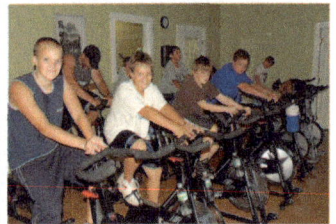

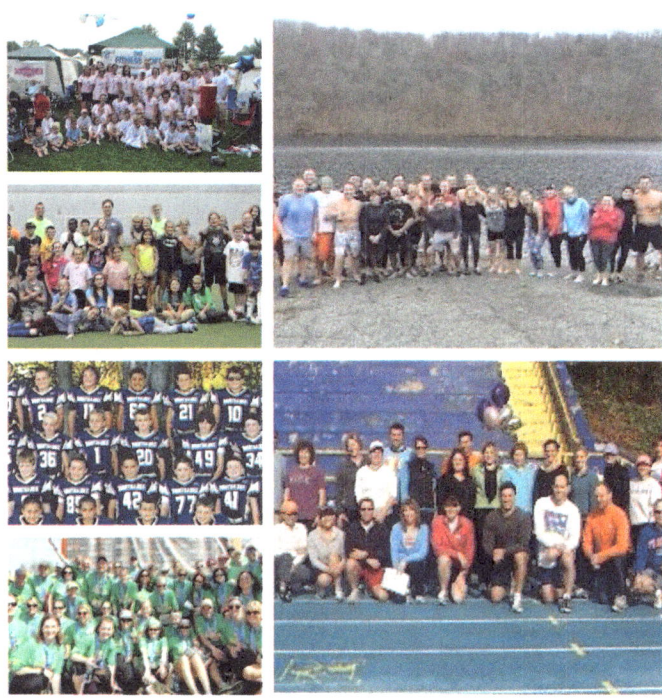
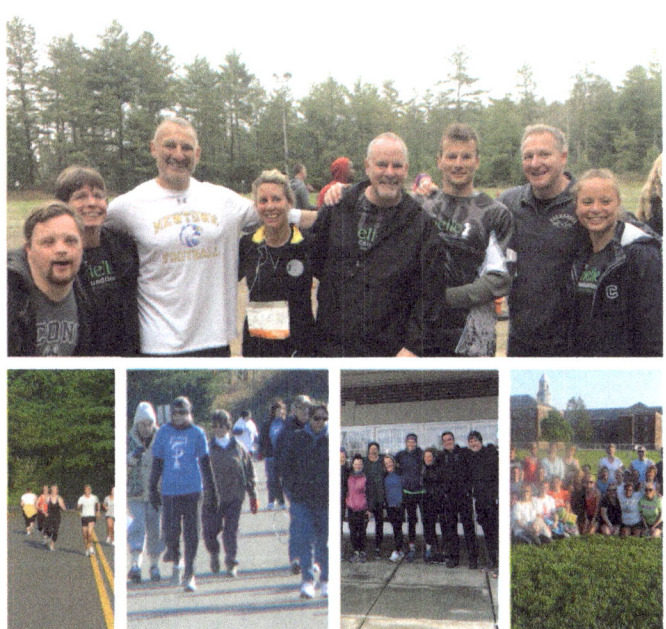

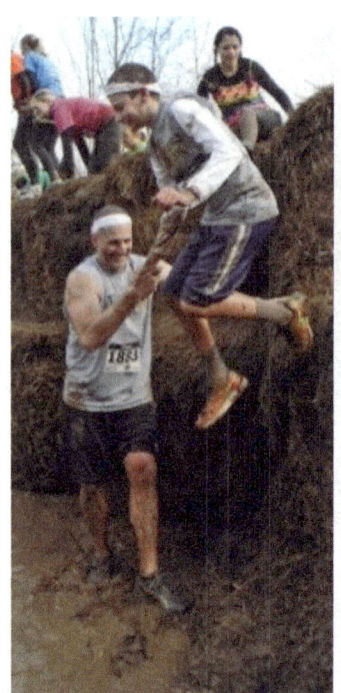
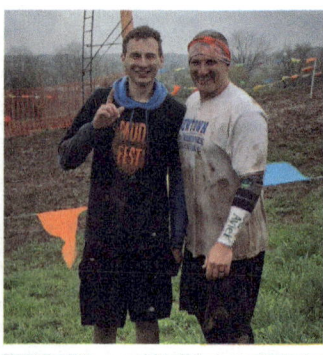
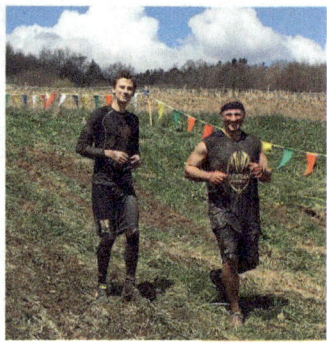
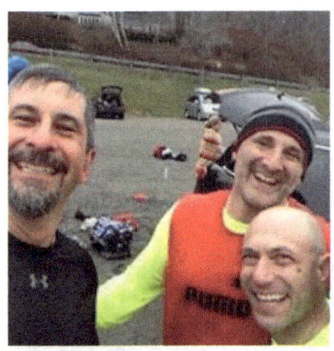
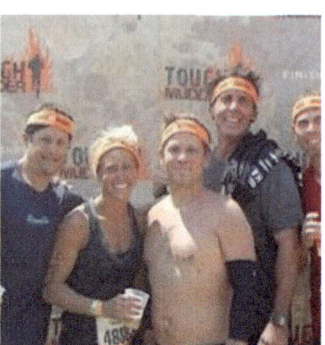
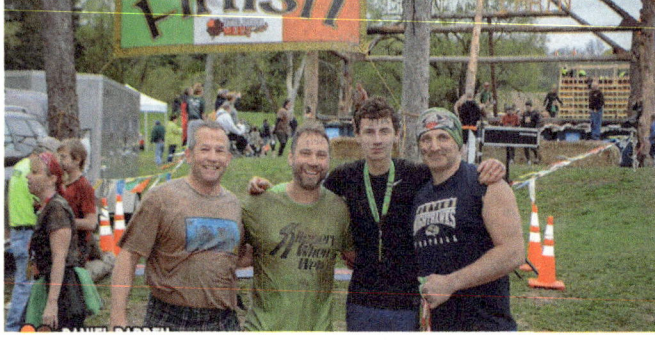

Chapter 9:
Your Mindset (contributions by Steve Gross)

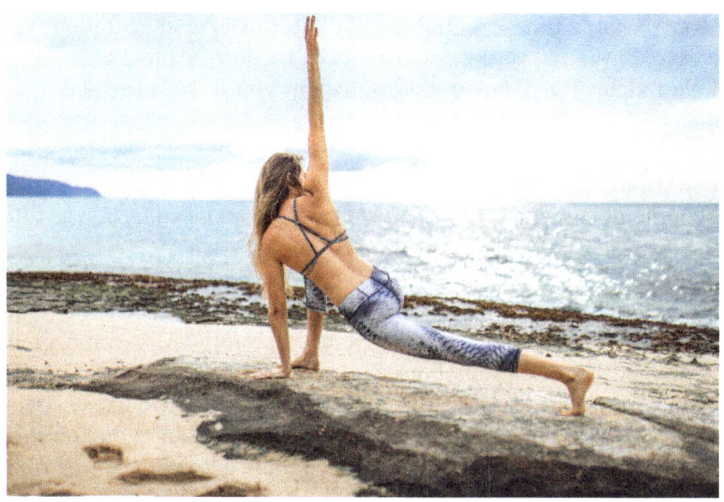

"What works best for you?"
As I've discussed throughout The Method, there are countless factors: hormonal, genetic, physical, environmental, financial, etc., which can greatly affect your wellness program. If you suffer from any medical, hormonal, emotional, or physical restrictions, please consult your physician to be best informed on how to proceed.

I personally don't believe these are reasons for failure, but opportunities to creatively find solutions. My background in sports medicine has taught me that there are so many ways to overcome restrictions and limitations. I have provided very effective workouts to individuals who were faced with physical, financial, and or time limitations. The key is staying positive and arming yourself with the necessary information to adjust your plan so that you can find success regardless of the issue.

Joint pain and physical restriction. There is a science behind learning how to stretch, strengthen, and avoid movements that will exacerbate a condition. Just knowing subtle technique adjustments can make a significant difference, but you need to seek information from a qualified health professional. For example, those looking to strengthen their knee by using a machine leg extension often don't realize they are putting significant stress on their knee joint by performing this movement. This exercise is poorly designed and doesn't account for stress forces at the knee joint. This isn't a matter of common sense though and is counter-intuitive for most people, but the end result is pain, frustration, and sometimes derailing a program.

Financial limitations. You can create an effective wellness program with basic resistance chords and open space. Granted this equipment can limit your ability to perform more advanced movements, but it is more than adequate to start a fitness routine. And I know that personal training can be expensive, but if you change your mindset to view health and wellness as an investment, I believe the information you'll be provided will be invaluable.

Time limitations. While I appreciate that wellness is a time commitment, please remember that a very effective program can take place in as little as 30 minutes.

So you get the idea, you will face hurdles and challenges adhering to a life of wellness. I just provided some practical solutions to some of these problems and hopefully this book has provided scientific information on how to best navigate a successful wellness program, but I'd like to conclude by talking about your **mindset**. This is the one variable you control that provides a positive outcome when combined with the appropriate information.

As we conclude the book and transition into how to apply the Method Training Program, I'd like to share a unique perspective from a friend of mine, Steve Gross, on how a positive mindset can significantly impact your fitness program.

As a quick introduction, Steve Gross is the founder and chief playmaker of the Life is Good Kids Foundation and a highly sought out inspirational speaker. Steve's signature approach has been widely adapted across the country and throughout the world in response to the social and emotional needs of children deeply impacted by poverty, violence and illness. In addition to his work in the social sector, Steve has worked with many corporations such as Vertex Pharmaceuticals, Million Dollar Roundtable Club, and IBM to demonstrate how optimistic leaders can inspire people and organizations through times of change. At first, this may not seem like Steve's background qualifies him to contribute to a wellness book but Steve's success in helping people find joy, happiness and optimism, driven by changing their mindset, is truly incredible. What's interesting is that I've worked with him in the past on some amazing community projects but didn't initially realize that his approach to 'mindset' could be the missing link for success in wellness for so many people.

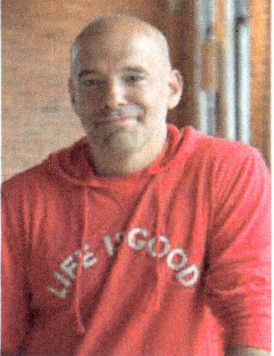

Founder and Chief Playmaker of the Life is Good Kids Foundation.

Steve suggests that if we're intentional in what we are doing and have a positive mindset, we can both prepare ourselves better for success and help avoid potential trip falls that can derail a fitness program. According to Steve, "WE are always changing, you are going to change regardless. So be intentional with what you want and go get it".

Below are a few ways he suggests changing your mindset about fitness.

Step #1 Show Gratitude- Express your gratitude for the **"get to"**

Steve Gross and the inspiration behind 'crucible' goal setting, Jeremy Richman, co-founder of The Avielle Foundation, would both often use the line that a challenge is a "get to opportunity" vs a "have to". I can remember anytime I was preparing to face a major challenge like a Tough Mudder or Ragnar Relay, Jer would quickly change my mindset with the simple expression, "we get to do this". The wording is simple, but the mindset change is transformational. If you view every challenge as a burden or "have to", you'll most likely quickly burn out, get drained or resentful of the act. However, if you embrace a challenge and express gratitude and optimism for the mere fact that you actually can do the activity, you will completely change your perspective. Learning how to embrace gratitude for something you never considered to be thankful for is a powerful mindset evolution.

Gratitude example toward exercising:
- Draining Mindset - "I have to work out!"
- Or… Get To Mindset
    - I'm fortunate enough to have access to a gym or equipment to work out

- I have muscles and joints that work, that will allow me to workout
- I have a cardiovascular system that allows my body to perform exercise
- I can afford workout clothes and equipment
- I have access to information that can help me workout safely and effectively
- I have access to foods that will provide my body with nutrition to fuel my activities
- I have access to a comfortable bed that will allow my body to rest, recover and rejuvenate

Step #2 Be Joyful (or Bring Playfulness)

Let's find ways to make wellness more fun so that in turn, we enjoy it and have a more positive attitude toward what we are about to do. This mindset is in line with the popular quote "love what you do and do what you love". By approaching exercise from a playful perspective, we can find ways to enjoy the experience better. This will require planning, but if we improve the experience, we will improve the outcome.

Examples of ways to make exercise more joyful:
- Create a play list
- Meet a friend
- Buy workout apparel that will make you feel better
- Take your workout to a scenic location
- Include healthy activities, sports and or games like playing frisbee vs using a stationary bike
- Plan an enjoyable, tasty post workout meal in advance as a healthy reward

Step #3 Define your Why (Y)

Knowing **Y** you are doing a particular exercise or workout will help you to create and better understand your value for exercising. Consequently, the experience will become much more intentional. The deeper you dive into the Y you are doing something, the more clarity you should achieve toward the true intent behind that activity. Once this value is understood, you'll better understand that exercise is really about living your best life.

For some people this is easier than for others. A parent wanting to improve their health so they can engage more actively with their kids and model a behavior their children can follow in their lives is a quality "Y" goal.

An adult looking to improve their health after developing signs of osteoporosis or early onset of diabetes are examples of clear and powerful "Y"'s. All of these examples have definable goals and accountability. However, it's not always that straightforward and you might have to really work and identifying your "Y". Steve suggests a simple exercise where you simply tag a question of "What would that goal do" once you accomplished it. Repeat this question and keep challenging yourself till you chip away and ultimately discover what's really lying below the surface.

For example, what if your goal is to look good in a bathing suit. At first glance this might seem like a shallow goal, but if pressed further, you might get a different outcome.
- Question -What would looking better in a bathing suit look like?
  - Answer- Feel better about yourself
- Question- What would that lead to?
  - More confidence
- Question- What would that lead to?
  - Able to pursue different opportunities
- Question- What would that lead to?
  - Feeling fulfilled in your career

This is a made-up scenario, but the value is "more than looking good in a bathing suit". This example is about confidence. You ultimately want to work out to gain more confidence. What would your life look like with more confidence? Steve challenges us to discover what is the true reason that we are doing this and that once we understand our Y, we can be more intentional with how we achieve it.

Step #4 Be Optimistic and Celebrate the Victories

Very often people don't see the gains, they only see where they struggle and consequently, don't see the victories. It's a normal condition to be highly self-critical. That doesn't make you overly sensitive, it makes you human and is a predisposed condition we all experience. Rick Hanson said it best, "our brains are negative magnets and Teflon for positive". So how you approach perceived failure is a significant mindset change. Focus on finding the positives in the process and DON'T ALLOW SELF CRITICAL THINKING TO derail you. This is a long-term, lifestyle change. As an example, a micro success like losing a 1/2 pound per month might be viewed as a failure if your goal was to lose more weight. However, from a macro perspective, you are on track to lose 6 pounds by the end of the year. So remember to STAY THE COURSE.

For more information on Steve's organization please visit https://www.lifeisgood.com/kidsfoundation/kidsfoundation.html.

So as you move forward with your wellness plan, remember in advance that your brain may trigger you to feel like you are failing, but a positive mindset will in fact remind you that you are succeeding and keep you on track towards even greater success!

Now let's move past any restrictions or excuses and let's build solutions!

One of the greatest strengths of The Method is creating individualized programs based on your strengths and weaknesses. **Behavior modification is hard, but it's much more effective when your initial steps allow you to focus on what you are good at, what you enjoy eating, and what is manageable.** It's also important to factor in physical restrictions which can potentially derail a wellness program if not identified. Your program has to be modified according to any limitations. Lastly, while there is some flexibility with goal setting and baseline measurements, these are very important components of a successful plan.

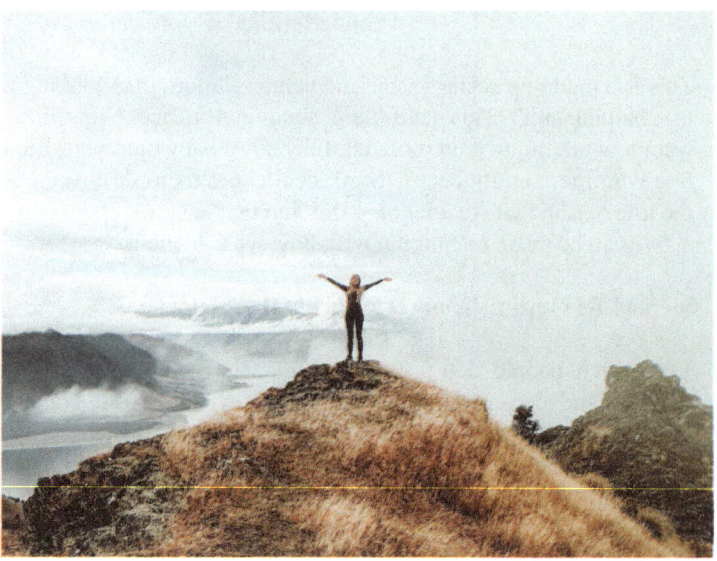

Chapter 10:
Building Your Plan

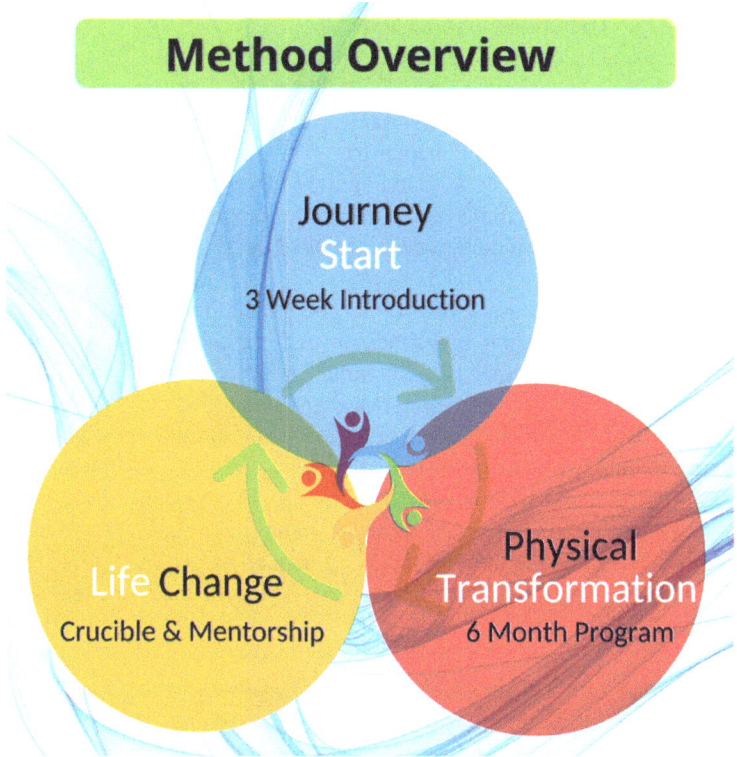

Your *Wellness Journey* is broken into **3 phases**:

1. **Journey Start -** 3 week introduction
   Your goal is to incorporate the 3 areas of wellness (nutrition, cardiovascular training, and strength training) into a safe, manageable, and accountable program.

2. **Physical Transformation -** 6 month program
   During this phase, your focus is on The Method Training Program and challenging your body, mind, and soul with a well-rounded, scientifically validated plan. Documenting your program and being

consistent will be key components as you build your body and the habits necessary for a life of health and wellness.

3. **Life Change**
During this final phase, you will further what you have accomplished throughout the Method Training Program and apply that to reaching your crucible and further, to mentoring someone else along their journey. Life is bigger than just getting in better shape, as you enter this phase, we want to awake the dreamer in you and have your successes inspire someone else.
   a. **Crucible Goal** (Chapter 7)
   Once you have found general levels of wellness success and sustainability, you will be pushed to create and train for a more significant goal.
   b. **Mentorship** (Chapter 8)
   Once you have found your own personal wellness success, we encourage you to mentor or support someone else to help them achieve their own success.

Regardless of your fitness level, you're encouraged to follow this step-by-step approach to building a wellness plan. The (new) area of wellness selected during a particular week or time period will be the main area of focus during that period. You are always encouraged to be as active and as healthy as possible, but we want to take small, measurable steps as we build an entire plan to establish behavioral change. Therefore, you can't advance from one area to the next without completing your current phase goal. If you address other areas (do more) at the same time, that's great, but your ability to advance to the next section is predicated on achieving the set goal of that particular phase. See below for an overview of the progression plan.

Sample Wellness Program

Pre Assessment – Journey Start
Sarah Smith is a 48-year-old female. She is 5'4" and weighs 155lbs with 26% body fat. Sarah's fitness level has declined over the years in part due to the time constraints of her life and by her body seemingly not working the way it used to. In addition to a demanding job, Sarah is also raising 3 kids with her husband. She's put on weight and feels deconditioned compared to her younger years when she was an active tennis player and loved running. Due to her current condition and some shoulder tendonitis, her activity levels, as well as nutrition, haven't been consistent. She's attempted, but unfortunately failed multiple times at finding a plan that will work for her to maintain. Sarah is frustrated and doesn't feel great

about the way she looks or feels. She's worked hard her entire life and is frustrated with her self-perceived failures in fitness.

Sarah receives a pre-assessment from a medical professional and is cleared to work out. She was advised to address her shoulder tendonitis by either seeing a physical therapist or certified personal trainer who understands how to address rotator cuff tendonitis.

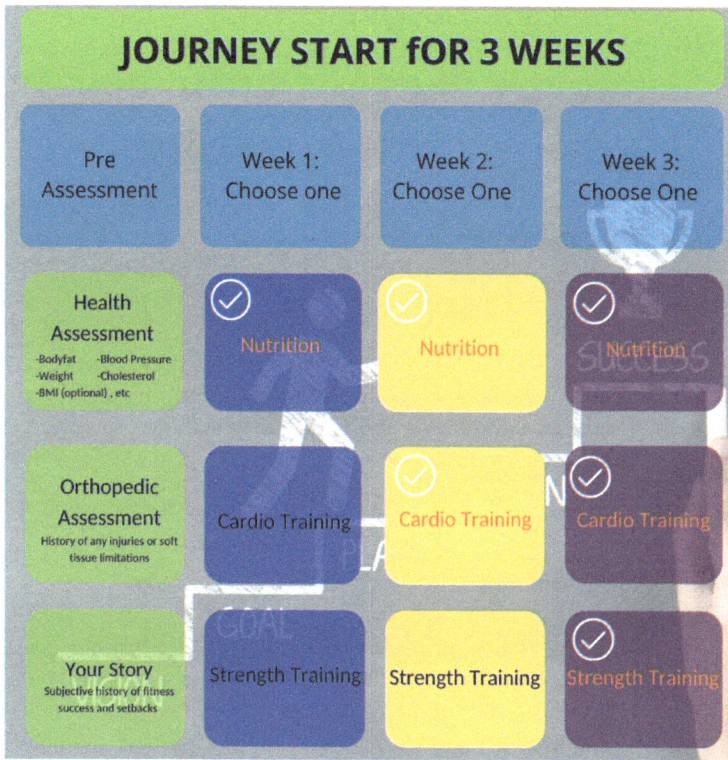

Week 1 - Journey Start
- She chooses **nutrition** as her week 1 goal.
- She tracks everything she is eating, drinks more water and focuses on smaller complete meals.

Week 2 – Journey Start
- After successfully addressing nutrition for a full week, Sarah chooses **cardio training** as her week 2 activity goal.
- She introduces more HIIT training and engages in three days of spinning. She enjoyed spin in the past and likes the accountability of attending class where she knows other people.

- As an additional cardiovascular activity, she attempts to walk her dogs in the park two additional days.
- She maintains her nutritional habits established during week 1 and also incorporates more fruits and vegetables throughout the day.

Week 3 – Journey Start
- Sarah adds **strength training** to her program for her last week of her **Journey Start**.
- She meets with a certified personal trainer twice a week who not only helps her learn the correct way to perform strength training movements, but is also helping her strengthen her rotator cuff and guides her in exercises that won't further aggravate that joint.
- To account for the additional days of strength training, she reduces spin class to one day a week.
- She is maintaining her nutritional habits from weeks 1 and 2.

By the start of week 4 Sarah has successfully completed the **Journey Start** phase and feels comfortable incorporating nutrition, cardiovascular training and strength training into her life. She is feeling healthier, has lost a few pounds and is feeling confident about entering the next phase, **Physical Transformation.**

Physical Transformation –

Over the next 6 months Sarah is committed to meeting with a trainer twice a week and training one day on her own. She splits her HIIT cardiovascular training between a spin class and boxing class. She continues to focus on her nutrition and is able maintain the habits she established during the Journey Start phase. She's eating cleaner foods that provide her with more energy to fuel her workouts like fruits, vegetables and lean proteins. The increased water intake and frequent quality meals have helped curb her appetite and increase her energy. She acknowledges that while she doesn't necessarily enjoy it, the tracking of both her nutrition and fitness activities throughout the week is a great resource for her and makes her accountable and able to stick to the plan.

PHYSICAL TRANSFORMATION for 6 Months

A — Month 1
4 week program performed 2-4 X's per week

Output variables should increase weekly

B — Month 2
Perform baseline re-evaluation

Significantly modify program from previous block

4 week program performed 2-4 X's per week

Output variables should increase weekly

C — Month 3
Significantly modify program from previous block

4 week program performed 2-4 X's per week

Output variables should increase weekly

D — Month 4
Perform baseline re-evaluation

Significantly modify program from previous block

4 week program performed 2-4 X's per week

Output variables should increase weekly

E — Month 5
Significantly modify program from previous block

4 week program performed 2-4 X's per week

Output variables should increase weekly

F — Month 6
Perform baseline re-evaluation

Significantly modify program from previous block

4 week program performed 2-4 X's per week

Output variables should increase weekly

Post Assessment
Perform a thorough evaluation matching your Journey Start

If you have achieved measurable success, advance to **Life Change** phase

If you haven't achieved success, go back to **Block E**

At the end of her 6-month fitness journey, Sarah's lost 12 pounds and reduced her bodyfat by 5%. She is sleeping better, happier, and more confident. She's also started playing tennis again recreationally on the weekends. She's thinking about what her crucible should be and thinks she wants to start running again and will train for a 5k with the hopes of running a half marathon and eventually a full marathon as her **Crucible Goal**.

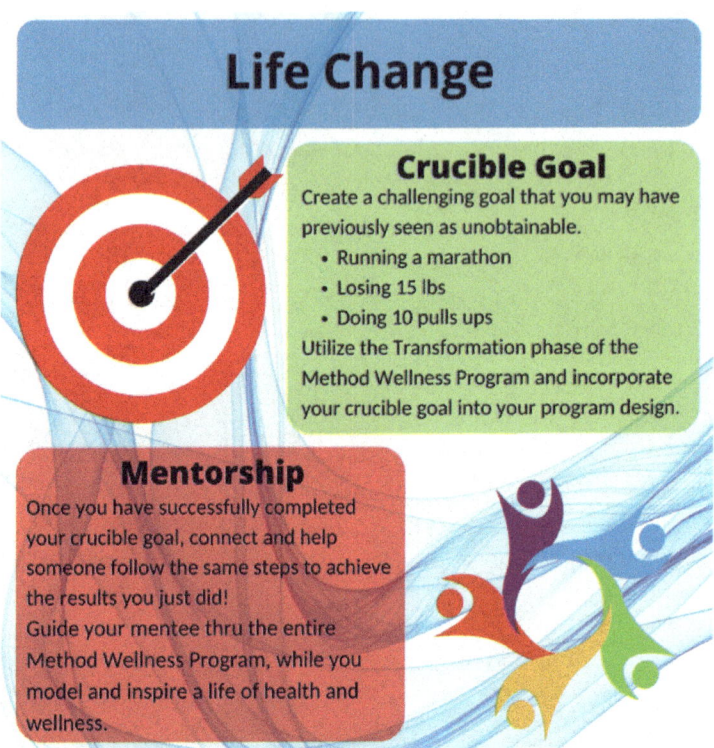

To better plan for her eventual goal of running a marathon, Sarah will meet with a running coach once a month in addition to meeting with a trainer once a week. Both professionals are assisting to design her a program to safely help her in the training required. As a result, Sarah is able to incorporate distance training into her overall program while still maintaining her nutritional adjustments and one to two days of HIIT training.

Maybe more importantly, Sarah's also entering the last phase of the Method Program by starting to **Mentor** others. She set up a free running group in her town and is coordinating a weekend run for all levels and types of runners. She shared her story on Facebook and made sure that anyone interested in participating knew that this was more about inclusion than performance. Participants range in their ability and experience. Sarah's fitness performance continues to grow and now with the accountability of a crucible goal and inspiring others in the process, she is truly on an amazing journey of connection and growth.

My Journey Packet

Assessment & Baseline Measurements

We will utilize information obtained during this thorough assessment to safely and effectively build your custom wellness plan. This assessment will also allow us to measure results and either validate the program or make necessary adjustments to improve it.

Nutrition and Activity Planner

We will use this as a journal and planner to account for your weekly nutritional intake and activity. Documenting your program is a key component of creating accountability and behavioral changes.

Workout Plan

We will use this to provide structure and guidance in executing the strength training component of your wellness plan.

The Method Training Program Assessment

Sarah Smith 07/14/20

Health Assessment

Body Composition	Pre-Assessment	Month 2	Month 4	Month 6	Post-Assessment
Height (Inches)	5' 4"	5' 4"	5' 4"		
Weight (Pounds)	155	152	148		
Body Fat %	26%	25%	22%		

Vitals / Cardiovascular	Pre-Assessment	Month 2	Month 4	Month 6	Post-Assessment
Resting Blood Pressure	120/80	120/80			
Resting Heart Rate	72	72			
Cholesterol	91/65				

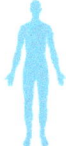

Orthopedic Assessment

Muscular Skeletal Assessment

Muscle	Stretch	Strengthen	Avoid	Skeletal Notes
external rc (teres minor)	x		Overhead Tennis Serve	Right Rotator Cuff Tendonitis, exasperated by tennis overhead serve. No apparent issue with metatrsal fracture but will monitor if any issues during weight bearing cardiovascular training.
internal rc (teres major)		x		
psoas major	x			

Injury History

Muscular Skeletal Injury History

Injury History	Treatment	Current Status
Right 2nd Metarsal fracture	physical therapy and reduced	Non issue

Your Story

What objective (measurable metrics) goals do you have?	subjective (self-reflective/how you want to feel and
I want to regain my body and get in better shape. I hope to lose 10 lbs and feel better about myself.	more energy and be able to engage with my family cognize who I am physically and hate how I appear ures.

What is your "Y"?	What are you... or what is stopping you?
I want to be happier and feel better about myself. I want to enjoy using my body again.	I don't have the time th... to exercise and my shoulder causes me pain o... ements. Otherwise, I

What wellness related activities are you currently doing?	What strategies and/or activities have worked for you in the past and why?
I used to love playing tennis and would like to make that part of my wellness plan again.	I was in the best shape of my life when I played tennis competitvely in high school and college. The joy of playing a sport that I loved and the motivation to get better lead to me getting in great shape.

Fitness Assessment

Muscular Strength	Pre-Assessment	Month 2	Month 4	Month 6	Post-Assessment
Bench Press	55 1RM	65 1RM	75 1RM		
Squat	NA				
Leg Press	155lbs 1RM	175lbs 1RM	195lbs 1RM		
Other					

Power & Aerobic Notes

Sarah presents with good overall strength and baseline cardiovascular capacity.

Muscular Endurance	Pre-Assessment	Month 2	Month 4	Month 6	Post-Assessment
Push-Ups	12	15	18		
Sit Up Test	22	25	28		
Plank Holds	35s	45s	58s		
Other					

Cardiovascular Endurance	Pre-Assessment	Month 2	Month 4	Month 6	Post-Assessment
Step Test	n/a				
EKG (add note)	n/a				
1.5 mile test	18.02	17.30	16.38		

Assessment Summary

Former college level tennis player who experienced dramatic reduction in excercise due to time constraints from both working and raising a family. The lack of activity spiraled into poor eating and becoming deconditioned and gaining weight. She has access to a gym and seasonal tennis courts. Sarah has a tendonitis in her R RC but with RC strengthening and modifying her serve we hope to reintroduce tennis as part of her wellness plan. She enjoys running and has some experience with basic strength training. We will introduce a modified running program and revisit and negate impact as she hasn't actively run in a few years. Nutrition will be focused with an initial goal of reducing late night sugary snacks and to eat more balanced meals. Once Sarah has established her cardio and strength program we will further focus on her nutritional intake and habits.

The Method Wellness and Nutritional Log

Nutrition	Sunday	Monday	Tuesday	Wednesday	Thursday	Friday	Saturday
Breakfast	Muesix						
Fruit	Banana	-	-	-	-	-	-
Snack (fruit)	Avocado	-	-	-	-	-	-
Lunch Protein	Salmon	-	-	-	-	-	-
Lunch Carb	Brown Rice	-	-	-	-	-	-
Lunch Vegetable	Salad	-	-	-	-	-	-
Snack (protein)	Almond	-	-	-	-	-	-
Dinner Protein	Duck	-	-	-	-	-	-
Dinner Carb	Barley	-	-	-	-	-	-
Dinner Veg	Broccoli	-	-	-	-	-	-
Dessert	-	-	-	-	-	-	-
or Fruit	Goji berries	-	-	-	-	-	-
Activity	Recreational Cardio	Strength	Long Low Intensity Cardio	Strength	High Cardio	Active Recovery	Strength
Choices	hiking	-	-	-	-	-	-

Notes:

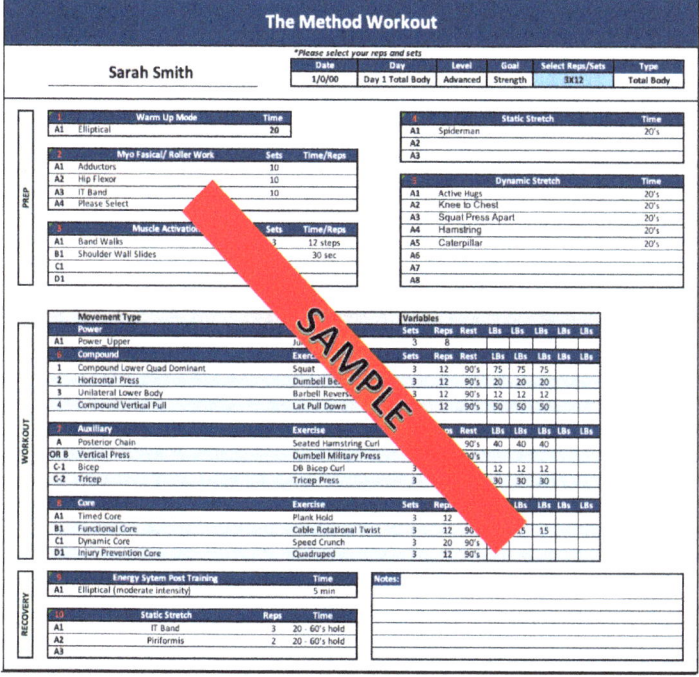

Tribe Community Wellness Programs and Services

The Method Training Program reflects the science and experience of years of personal training and is the epicenter of my company, Tribe Community Wellness (TCW). TCW is committed to empowering communities and individuals to achieve wellness while also connecting with each other through various programs and services.

These programs include:

- Private Training and Group Training
- Online- Virtual Training
- Family Adventure Races
- Afterschool Programs
- Corporate and Municipal Wellness Consulting
- Home Gym Design

If you would like to learn more about any of these services or programs or would like to offer feedback, please reach out to me at:

tribecommunitywellness@gmail.com
www.tribecommunitywellness.com

About the Author

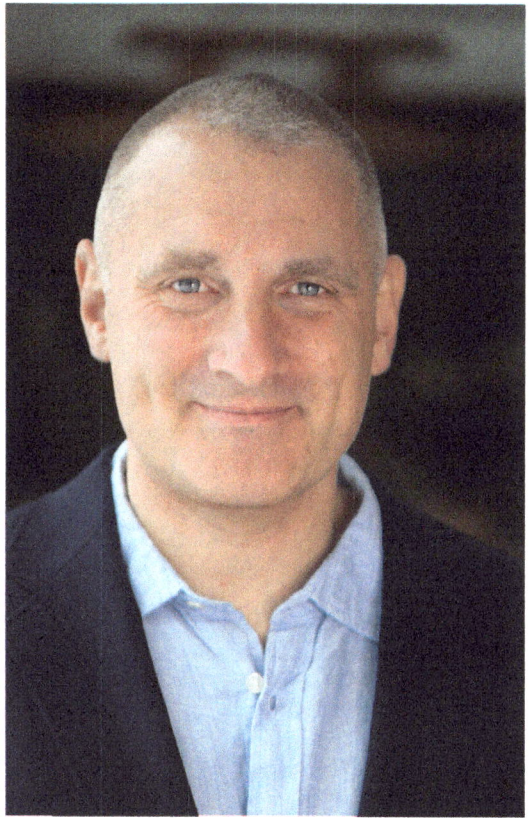

Cody Foss -- M.S., L.A.T.C., C.S.C.S., P.E.S.
With almost 30 years of experience and having obtained the highest level of academic and professional certifications, I have been recognized as an established expert in the field of health and wellness. I have owned and managed health clubs and sports medicine facilities in NYC and Fairfield County, CT. In addition to providing wellness or rehabilitation programs for hundreds of children, I have had the privilege of working with Olympic and professional athletes. I have been published in multiple magazines and newspapers and have enjoyed the opportunity to speak on many topics related to health and wellness. I have created and assisted in several community wellness engagements, working collaboratively with multiple local and national organizations.

In addition to wellness-based programs, I have also developed several community programs, including the Spark Afterschool Program for The Avielle Foundation. The Spark Afterschool Program embeds my personal belief that social isolation amongst children is not acceptable. Culturally enriched communities create greater opportunities for peer connections. All children need to learn how to take care of themselves physically, socially, and emotionally. Lastly, that communities should be defined by their ability to demonstrate compassion, empathy, and support of one another.

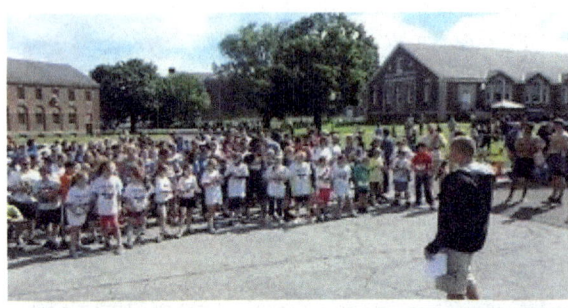

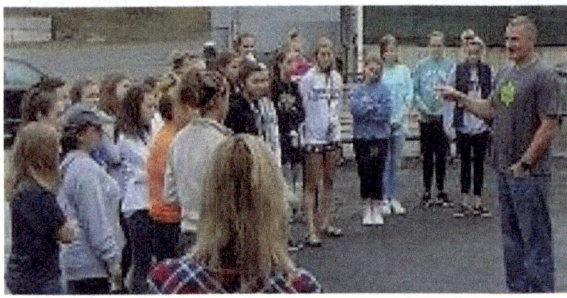

Top: Speaking to race participants in Newtown, CT.
Bottom: Speaking to a local lacrosse team.

My "Y" is simple. *I feel like a better human being when I'm helping others.* This emotion is further enhanced when more people are involved in this process and collectively we form our "tribe".

My life reflects a constant search in helping others. From my roots in sports medicine and fitness, to evolving large scale community initiatives, I have been building my tribe my entire life. This book reflects my personal and professional experiences in this process and provides a resource for anyone looking to better their health and wellness in a sustainable, inspirational, and proven way!

Articles Written: Cody has contributed or written articles for the following magazines/ newspapers:
- Redbook Magazine
- The Newtown Bee
- The News-Times

- The Ridgefield Press
- Shape Magazine
- The Review Magazine
- Westchester Magazine

Lectures: Cody has performed over a dozen lectures and seminars on various topics including:
- ACL prevention strategies for the female athlete (Hospital for Special Surgery)
- Performance Strategies for Baseball
- Dynamic Stretching and Speed Drills for Football
- Performance, Nutrition and Injury Prevention Strategies for Dancers
- Prevention of Lower Back Pain
- Physical Programming Strategies for Physical Education Instructors
- The 5 Biggest Myths in the Fitness Industry
- Why We are Failing at Fitness and What You Need to Know to Change It

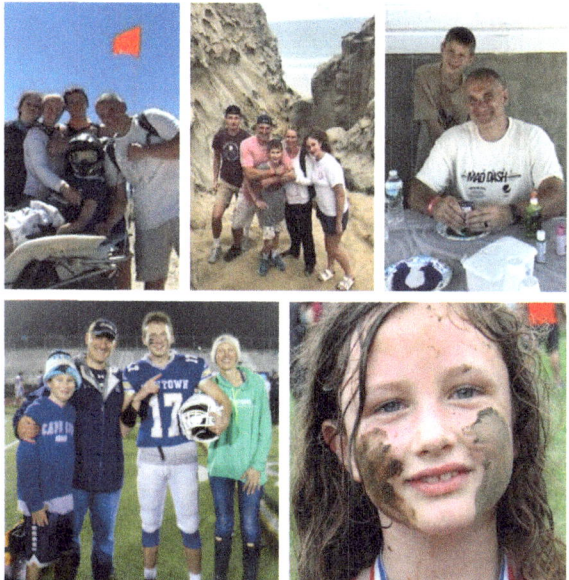

Athletes Cody has trained:
- NFL Athletes
- Olympic Athletes
- Champion Tae Kwon Do Athletes
- US Athletic Training Center
- The Spence School

- Knicks City Dancers
- Professional Boxers
- Women's Professional Volleyball Association
- Manhattan College Basketball
- Division I and III Football Players
- Members of the 2005 National American Football Youth Football Champions
- Pee-Wee Hockey #2 in the state
- Ridgefield H.S. 2006 Varsity Hockey Team
- Nationally and State Ranked Figure Skaters
- FCIAC All-Section Baseball
- FCIAC All Section Softball
- FCIAC All Section Basketball
- Multiple Varsity Athletes
- Men's Soccer
- Women's Soccer
- Women's Lacrosse
- Men's Lacrosse
- Hockey
- Women's Basketball
- Women's Field Hockey
- Swimming
- Equestrian
- NHS Football
- NHS Girls Softball
- NHS TENNIS
- NHS GIRLS LACROSSE
- NHS BOYS LACROSSE
- NHS BOYS HOCKEY
- AYF FOOTBALL NEWTOWN

Current Work Experience:
- Northeast Regional Manager of The Ben's Bells Project, Newtown, CT
    - Oversee all Operations in Northeast
    - Community Outreach
    - Public Speaking
- Owner of Tribe Community Wellness, Newtown, CT
    - Multi-dimensional wellness company providing community wellness events, health & wellness business consulting, and life wellness plan consulting.
- Creator and Director of the Spark Afterschool Program, Newtown CT
- Creator and Director of the Mad Dash Adventure Race, Newtown CT
- Community Volunteer

- Youth Football Coach
- The Avielle Foundation & Ben's Lighthouse

Former Work Experience:
- Director of NYA Sports and Fitness Center, Newtown, CT
- Owner of The Fitness Loft, Newtown, CT
- Director of Performance Programs at the Ridgefield Fitness Club, Ridgefield, CT
- Head Athletic Trainer and Strength Coach at the Spence School, NYC
- Highest Ranked Trainer at Equinox and New York Health and Racquetball Club, NYC
- Manager, Athletic Trainer and Strength Coach at the US Athletic Training Center, NYC

Collaborative Partners and influences:
- The Avielle Foundation
- Playmakers

Bibliography

"All About Muscle Growth." *Precision Nutrition*, 11 Feb. 2013, www.precisionnutrition.com/all-about-muscle-growth.

Brooke, et al. "One Pound Of Fat Versus One Pound Of Muscle: Clearing Up The Misconceptions -." *BambooCore Fitness*, 7 Nov. 2017, www.bamboocorefitness.com/one-pound-of-fat-versus-one-pound-of-muscle-clearing-up-the-misconception/.

Davis, Jeanie Lerche. "Get More Burn From Your Workout." *WebMD*, www.webmd.com/fitness-exercise/features/get-more-burn-from-your-workout#1/.

Fife, Bruce. *The Stevia Deception: The Hidden Dangers of Low-Calorie Sweeteners*. Piccadilly Books, Ltd., 2017.

Filingeri, Vincent S. *Fat Control: The NET Equation*. First Edition Design Pub., 2011.

Grant, Bob. "Fat Cell Numbers Fixed in Adults." *The Scientist: Exploring Life, Inspiring Innovations*, 4 May 2008, www.the-scientist.com/the-nutshell/fat-cell-numbers-fixed-in-adults-45166/.

Iliades, Chris. "7 Ways Strength Training Boosts Your Health and Fitness." *Everyday Health, Inc.*, 13 May 2019, www.everydayhealth.com/fitness/add-strength-training-to-your-workout.aspx/.
Accessed 5 May 2020.

Kent, Linda Tarr. "A Pound of Fat Vs. a Pound of Muscle." *LIVESTRONG.COM*, Leaf Group, 11 Sept. 2017, www.livestrong.com/article/438693-a-pound-of-fat-vs-a-pound-of-muscle/.

Kinucan, Paige, and Len Kravitz. "Controversies in Metabolism." *The University of New Mexico*, www.unm.edu/~lkravitz/Article folder/metabolismcontroversy.html.

Matthews, Jessica. "Why Is the Concept of Spot Reduction Considered a Myth?" *Ace Fitness*, September 2009, www.acefitness.org/education-and-resources/lifestyle/blog/44/why-is-the-concept-of-spot-reduction-considered-a-myth/.

McCoy, Krisha. "Can Eating Too Few Calories Stall Your Metabolism?" *Everyday Health*, 3 April 2009, www.everydayhealth.com/weight/fewer-calories-stalls-metabolism.aspx.

Nall, Rachel. "How to Increase Your Metabolism." *Medical News Today*, 12 Oct. 2018, www.medicalnewstoday.com/articles/323328.
"Obesity." *University of California San Francisco Benioff Children's Hospital*. www.ucsfbenioffchildrens.org/conditions/obesity/.

"Obesity In Children And Teens." *AACAP*, no. 79, April 2016, www.aacap.org/aacap/families_and_youth/facts_for_families/fff-guide/obesity-in-children-and-teens-079.aspx.

Olson, Michele Ph.D. "Tabata: It's a HIIT!." *ACSM's Health & Fitness Journal*, vol. 18, no. 5, September/October 2014.

Raman, Ryan. "Why Your Metabolism Slows Down With Age." *Healthline*, 24 September 2017, www.healthline.com/nutrition/metabolism-and-age.

Schoenfeld, Brad, and Jay Dawes. "High-Intensity Interval Training: Applications for General Fitness Training." *Strength and Conditioning Journal*, vol. 31, no. 6, December 2009.

St. Pierre, Brian. "Can Eating Too Little Actually Damage Your Metabolism?" *Precision Nutrition*, www.precisionnutrition.com/metabolic-damage. Accessed 5 May 2020.

"The 3500 Calorie Rule." *Bodyrecomposition*, www.bodyrecomposition.com/fat-loss/3500-calorie-rule.html/.

Volpi, Elena, et. al. "Muscle Tissue Changes With Aging." *PubMed Central*, 12 Jan. 2010, www.ncbi.nlm.nih.gov/pmc/articles/PMC2804956/.

West, Helen. "10 Easy Ways to Boost Your Metabolism (Backed by Science)." *Healthline*, 27 July 2018, www.healthline.com/nutrition/10-ways-to-boost-metabolism

Made in the USA
Columbia, SC
06 January 2023